D0663531

Stroke

Stroke

A Comprehensive Guide to "Brain Attacks" Everything You Need to Know

Dr. Vladimir Hachinski
Larissa Hachinski

JESSAMINE COUNTY PUBLIC LIBRARY
600 South Main Street
Nicholasville, KY 40356
(859) 885-3523

FIREFLY BOOKS

A FIREFLY BOOK

Published by Firefly Books (U.S.) Inc. 2003

Copyright © 2002 by Vladimir Hachinski and Larissa Hachinski

All rights reserved. No part of this publication may be reproduced, stored in a retrieval system or transmitted in any form or by any means, electronic, mechanical, photocopying, recording or otherwise, without the prior written permission of the Publisher.

First Printing

(U.S.) Publisher Cataloging-in-Publication Data
(Library of Congress Standards)

Hachinski, Vladimir.
   Stroke : A comprehensive guide to "brain attacks" everything you need to know / Vladimir Hachinski. – 1st ed.
[192] p. : ill. ; cm. (Your personal health)
Includes index. 3 2530 60562 7643
Summary: Understanding how strokes occur, their treatments, and the aftermath.
ISBN: 1-55209-642-4 (pbk.)
1. Cerebrovascular disease – Popular works. 2. Cerebrovascular disease – Treatment – Popular works. I. Title. II. Series.
616.81 21   RC388.5.H33   2003

Published in the United States in 2003 by
Firefly Books (U.S.) Inc.
P.O. Box 1338, Ellicott Station
Buffalo, New York, USA
14205

616.81
H ACH

Published in Canada in 2002 by Key Porter Books Limited.

Design: Peter Maher
Electronic formatting: Heidy Lawrance Associates

Printed and bound in Canada

Contents

Acknowledgments

No book is an accomplishment of the authors alone. We are grateful to the patients whose stories inspired several of the illustrative vignettes. Many other people gave their precious time to help us create this concise guide. They were interviewed, provided material or reviewed segments of the book and we are most appreciative of their efforts. For their valued contributions, we thank Dr. J. Paul Caldwell, Dr. Ashok Devasanapathy, Dr. Hillel Finestone, Connie Frank, Dr. Donald Lee, Cheryl Mayer, Dr. Harold Merskey, Christine O'Callaghan, Breeda O'Farrell, Joanna Pierazzo, Jeanette Rewucki, Dr. Brian Silver, Dr. Arturo Tamayo and Dr. Robert Teasell.

Finally, this was a family affair. My father has been a constant inspiration and teacher. I have always admired his quest for answers and am honored to be part of his work. My mother, Mary Ann Hachinski, has been a loving and wise influence to all. And to my husband, Douglas Keddy, who was always ready with an editing pen and an open heart: thank you.

Larissa Hachinski

Foreword

Since my childhood, I have been aware of the impressive power of medicine. As a girl, and now as a young woman, I have watched my father and his colleagues in their untiring quest to prevent and lessen the damage caused by strokes, or "brain attacks"—a term my father introduced to stress the need to treat stroke with the same urgency as heart attacks. Brain attack and stroke are the same thing. A brain attack or stroke occurs when part of the brain suddenly stops working, because of a blocked or burst blood vessel.

A stroke can be a devastating event, but luckily the story does not end there. Over the years, my father has seen many changes in the treatment of stroke patients. When he first started his medical career, there was a lot of uncertainty and fear about stroke. Now, much has improved. People can play an important role in protecting themselves by recognizing the symptoms of brain attack and taking action. The sooner someone who has had a stroke gets medical attention, the better are the chances for recovery; stroke units that offer complete care are being set up across North America.

I am delighted that I can join my father's team and contribute to his life's work. He has been involved with neurology for over 30 years. For the past decade, he was the Richard and Beryl Ivey Professor and Chair of the Department of Clinical Neurological Sciences in London, Ontario, Canada, one of the leading centers in stroke treatment for more than three decades. Currently he is the editor-in-chief of *Stroke*, the leading publication in the field, is active in research and continues to see patients and to teach.

Our goal has been to create a book to educate and inform people about brain attack. Health professionals often forget how difficult it can be for non-experts to understand their jargon, and we have tried to present all the essential information in clear and accessible language. Using a series of interviews drawn from my father's many years of expertise, we were able to garner a great amount of material. My father edited, supplemented and guided the material and I researched and wrote. I also interviewed doctors, nurses, rehabilitation experts, caregivers and stroke survivors, all of whom took great care to explain their role in stroke treatment. Their contributions of medical expertise and human experience have enabled us to make this book a complete picture of stroke treatment in a time of great progress.

L.H.

Introduction

Suddenly, and often without warning, a life can change forever. In an instant, a blood vessel in the brain is blocked, or bursts, and part of the brain stops working. The consequences are immediate. Strokes spare no age, no gender, no ethnicity and no country. They are a leading cause of death and disability. Much can be done to prevent these tragedies, but only if the symptoms of stroke are recognized and heeded.

Stroke used to be called *apoplexy*, from a Greek word meaning "to strike down." The term *stroke* also implies being felled by fate. Some doctors still use the term *cerebrovascular accident*, or *CVA*, to describe stroke, but this is misleading because many strokes are not really accidents; they are preventable catastrophes. Many are predictable and more are treatable. Consider heart attacks. People know that chest pain can mean a threat to life, even though not all chest pains are related to a heart attack. But not everyone knows that sudden loss of vision, or of movement or feeling in a limb, may be caused by a stroke, or may be a warning sign of a stroke, and that anyone having these symptoms needs urgent medical attention. Yet it's essential that the onset of stroke be recognized and treated immediately.

Unlike the often painful symptoms of a heart attack, the warnings of stroke can be subtle, and the effects of the attack

> ## Strokes of genius
> The rich and famous are as vulnerable to brain attack as the poor and humble. A burst blood vessel ended the terror of the fierce conqueror Attila the Hun, and a blocked artery silenced the creative genius of the great Canadian pianist Glenn Gould. When United States President Woodrow Wilson and Prime Minister Winston Churchill of Great Britain had strokes, it affected not only them, but history. However, not all strokes are devastating. Louis Pasteur, the developer of the rabies vaccine, did his best work after suffering a stroke at the age of 47.

itself more lasting. Basic functions such as communicating, walking and thinking, as well as personality, may be changed. No stroke survivor, no survivor's caregiver, ever takes the simple things for granted again. The disease strikes at the core of our functioning and our being.

Together, strokes and heart attacks account for about three-quarters of all deaths in the United States and Canada. People often consider stroke a less serious problem than heart attack, but according to information from the Canadian Heart and Stroke Foundation and the U.S. National Stroke Association, stroke is the leading cause of adult disability in North America. In the United States, someone experiences a stroke every 45 seconds. Approximately four million Americans are living with the effects of stroke. In Canada, approximately 50,000 new cases occur each year, and at any given time about 200,000 Canadians are living with the aftereffects.

This is a very real social issue. Stroke affects not only the sufferer but also the family, friends, employers and taxpayers; not only the person but also the community. There are devastating emotional costs, and there are also economic ones. In North America, billions of dollars a year go to cover the direct and indirect expenses of stroke, including medical care, lost wages, pensions and drugs. The prevention of stroke is an important goal for society as well as for the individual.

What would happen to you if you became a victim of stroke? The Canadian Heart and Stroke Foundation has put together a profile of likely outcomes. Out of four people who have a stroke, one will recover fully, one will recover incompletely, one will remain disabled and may require assistance with the basics of living, and one will die. After the first stroke, all survivors have a 10 percent risk, each year, of having another. Don't allow yourself to be one of those numbers. If you take an active part in protecting yourself and your loved ones, you can make a real difference. The progress in stroke prevention and treatment in the past decade has been encouraging. Frequently, when the warning symptoms are recognized and quickly acted upon, the damage caused by stroke can be minimal. New technology, treatment and greater awareness are our greatest weapons in the battle. Educating yourself about stroke is the first step toward prevention.

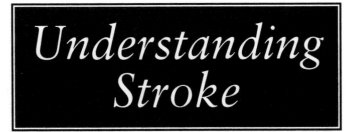

Understanding Stroke

A stroke, or brain attack, is a sudden loss of brain function that is caused when the blood supply to part of the brain has been disrupted. The effects of a stroke depend on the size and location of the brain area deprived of blood or damaged by blood. Knowing how the brain works and what each part does will help you understand why people may be unable to do certain things after a stroke.

Hippocrates, the father of medicine, observed 24 centuries ago that apoplexy (stroke) could lead to unconsciousness and coma, and concluded that the brain was the seat of consciousness. Later it was noted that if a stroke affected the left side of the brain the patient was paralyzed on the right side of the body, and vice versa. In the 1800s, the French scientist Paul Broca showed that a stroke in the front part of the left side of the brain caused loss of speech. The function that is lost when a particular part of the brain is damaged gives us clues to the normal role of that part of the brain. The brain is capable of remarkable recovery in the face of major damage.

The human brain is incredibly complex. It's made up of billions of nerve cells (*neurons*), each communicating with thousands of others, allowing us to think, move and live. The brain and the spinal cord together make up the body's central nervous system (CNS). The brain receives and sends signals from and to all parts of the body, from the tips of your fingers to the tips of your toes.

The nerve cells are in branching clusters on the surface (*cerebral cortex*) and the inside (*basal ganglia*) of the brain. Insulating material covers the large branches of nerves; these are the pathways along which messages are sent and received.

The brain itself is gray-pink in color, slightly soft in texture, and weighs about three pounds (1.4 kilos). It has several distinct areas, each responsible for a different part of our functioning.

Areas of the Brain: What They Do and How They May Be Affected

Brain Stem
The *brain stem* is nestled below the larger part of the brain; it is considered to be an extension of the spinal cord. The brain stem is responsible for the many vital automatic functions of the body, such as breathing, maintaining blood pressure and heart rate, swallowing, chewing, eye movements and quick reflexes—functions we don't give a second thought to as long as they are working smoothly. The brain stem is also home to the major passageways between the upper brain and the rest of the body. A stroke originating in this area may be fatal if it involves the vital centers. Luckily, most of the time only part of the brain stem is involved and life is spared. Double vision, imbalance, trouble swallowing, and weakness or numbness of the face or limbs may result, depending on the part of the brain stem affected.

Cerebellum
At the back of the brain stem sits the *cerebellum* ("little brain"), which coordinates movements and balance. It also stores the

memory of habitual muscle movements, such as the pattern of muscles used to swing a golf club or sweep the garage. A brain attack in the cerebellum causes unsteadiness, incoordination and clumsiness of the limbs involved.

Areas of the Brain

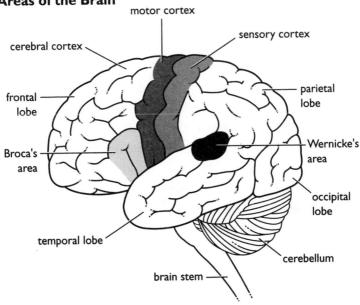

Cerebrum

The *cerebrum* (brain) defines us as humans. It receives information from all parts of the body, analyzes it, compares it with previously stored information and decides if any action needs to be taken; it then sends signals to the muscles, causing them to perform the appropriate actions. All of this happens almost instantaneously. This speed of operation is one of the reasons that the cerebrum is considered the most highly developed area of the brain.

The cerebrum has two halves, or hemispheres, the right and the left, each controlling the side of the body opposite to it.

While each hemisphere is specialized and controls certain general functions, the hemispheres are richly connected by nerve fibers that allow them to work together, and even to make up for each other.

The *right hemisphere* controls movements on the left side of the body. It also recognizes shapes, angles, proportions and visual patterns, including people's faces. It is important for musicality, creativity and imagination. The right hemisphere controls emotion and the sense of one's position in space— one's awareness of one's body. If it is damaged, people may no longer feel that their body is their own. People who are paralyzed on their left side may not recognize their own left hand.

The *left hemisphere* controls movements of the right side of the body. It also controls speech. It is considered to be the more logical hemisphere, responsible for analytical thought, problem-solving and language. A brain attack in the left hemisphere may result in paralysis on the right side of the body, and in problems communicating and understanding.

Each hemisphere of the cerebrum is further divided into four lobes. The *occipital lobe* is the center for vision. Individual signals gathered by the eyes are processed in these lobes. A stroke that damages the occipital lobes may leave a person blind, even though the eyes themselves remain unharmed.

The *temporal lobe* is where memories are formed and partly stored. The good news about the effect of stroke in this spot is that unless both the right and left temporal lobes are affected, memory loss is not likely to be permanent. It seems that the other temporal lobe, and other areas of the brain, are able to make up for the damaged area.

Other important functions of the temporal lobe are hearing and understanding speech. The area for understanding speech (*Wernicke's area*) spreads into the neighboring parietal lobe and is found in the left hemisphere in right-handed people and in two-thirds of left-handers. A stroke involving this area almost never affects hearing, but it does impair the person's ability to understand language.

Our sense of space and perspective, and our interpretation of our world, depend on the *parietal lobes*. These lobes also contain a strip of *sensory cortex*, which straddles the top of the brain and receives and interprets information from the body.

The *frontal lobes* are the most highly developed parts of the brain. Human frontal lobes are twice as large as those of other species such as apes. The frontal lobes shape behavior, anticipation, emotion and, most important, thinking. They are also vital for motor function, planning and the expression of language. The center for speech expression (*Broca's area*) is in the left frontal lobe of right-handers and of two-thirds of left-handers. Our ability to test the frontal lobe is limited, and the degree of impairment here is not always identified.

A stroke here can change personality, thinking and planning abilities—depending on what part of the frontal lobe is affected. It may be difficult for people to do tasks that require actions in sequence. They are usually able to take the first step but not to progress beyond it, because they forget what the next step is, or they cannot send the necessary messages to the muscles to complete the tasks. A complicated idea may be beyond their grasp.

The frontal lobe also houses the area of the brain where abstract thinking, initiative and social inhibitions reside. Stroke survivors who have damage in this area may lose their zest for living, or may become very impulsive in their behavior; unable to tell what is appropriate and what is not, some stroke survivors swear and say other socially unacceptable things.

If Broca's area is damaged, the person may be unable to speak (*Broca's expressive aphasia*). Most often he or she can utter sounds and simple words, such as "yes" or "damn."

It is not uncommon for stroke survivors who can hardly speak a word to be able to swear in frustration. Even if they didn't

The singing mute

In seventeenth-century Sweden, an apparent miracle occurred. A 33-year-old farmer's son had a violent illness that left him mute, and weak on the right side of the body. He could utter no word except "yes." But when he went to church, he joined in the singing with no difficulty! Skeptics thought he was faking, since he sang all the words of the hymns clearly but still did not speak. Others saw him as a freak. The faithful believed it was a miracle.

Now we know that he had probably had a stroke that affected the speech centers of the left side of the brain. The right brain has some capacity for language, but is much more involved in music and intonation.

swear before, they sometimes start to do so, to the distress of their families. Emotion can enable them to utter swearwords or other words expressing strong feeling. Singing "Happy Birthday" or some other well-known song often prompts them to carry on for a few lines. Some music therapists believe that such exercises speed recovery of speech. This is uncertain; what is certain is that these exercises encourage both the individual and his or her family, who can believe that "The words are there, you just need to learn to bring them out."

The *motor cortex* of the frontal lobe is a strip in front of the sensory cortex of the parietal lobe. If it is damaged, there may be paralysis of the face, arm or leg.

Because the human brain is such a delicate and complex organ, and is so central to our functioning, the effects of stroke can be devastating. Unlike other cells in our body, brain cells do not reproduce, so any brain cells that die during a stroke are lost forever. Recent research suggests, however, that parts of the brain can grow new cells. The death of various brain cells does not necessarily mean the end of the function they controlled. Other parts of the brain can eventually assume some of these functions. But this process involves relearning skills, and it takes time and patience.

T W O

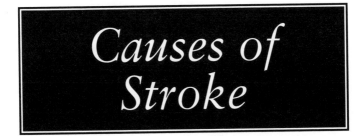

Causes of Stroke

Within the cells of our body, life is sustained through a constant process of combustion. The cells burn fuel, and—like a fire—they use up oxygen in the process. The main fuel for the cells is glucose, a form of sugar that we extract from food. Glucose (also called blood sugar) and oxygen are both transported around our bodies by our blood. If the flow of blood is disrupted, so is the supply of glucose and oxygen.

Although the brain makes up only 2 percent of our body weight, it consumes 20 percent of the oxygen in the blood to burn the glucose. Some organs of the body, such as the liver, can live on other substances, but the adult brain is continuously active, even during sleep, and it depends on a constant fresh supply of oxygen and glucose. Any interruption interferes with its function.

When part of the brain doesn't receive the blood and oxygen it needs, it is forced to get its energy by breaking down glucose without oxygen. This method is much less efficient, and it produces lactic acid, which is harmful to the brain. Having insufficient energy, the neurons can't send or receive messages, and chemical messengers between the neurons, called *neurotransmitters*, spill and do harm.

7

One of the most abundant neurotransmitters, glutamate, is also one of the most toxic. Unless the blood flow is restored, the cells' fine balance of vital elements such as potassium and calcium falters, cell membranes break down, inflammation flares and brain cells begin to die. The brain swells and the person's condition worsens.

How Blood Reaches the Brain

The brain is supplied by four arteries arranged in two systems, the *carotid* and the *vertebrobasilar*. The carotid arteries can be felt on each side of the neck, and carry most of the blood to the brain. At about the middle of the side of the neck, the common carotid artery divides into an internal carotid artery that goes to the brain and an external carotid artery that supplies the face and scalp. Where arteries branch into two, in a *bifurcation*, the dynamics of the blood flow change. This is often where hardening of the arteries (*atherosclerosis*), and narrowing of the arteries' interior, occur. The narrowing, known as *carotid stenosis*, accounts for about a quarter of all strokes in the Western world.

The two *vertebral* arteries also supply the brain. They run inside the spinal vertebrae (backbone) and join at the base of the brain to form a single *basilar* artery. They supply blood to the core of the brain, the cerebellum and the inner and back part of the hemispheres. This is the *vertebrobasilar system*, which deals with vital functions.

Once the arteries of the carotid and vertebrobasilar system reach the base of the brain, they join to form the *circle of Willis*. If one of the four main arteries supplying the brain is closed off, enough blood will usually come through the circle of Willis to make up the difference. Similarly, branches of the carotid and vertebral arteries and branches of the main arteries of the brain itself can connect and offer *collateral circula-*

tion to an area deprived of blood. The main threat to the brain comes not from the narrowing or even closing of the carotid arteries, which collateral circulation can often compensate for, but from blood clots that form on the roughened surface of the narrowings and are then carried away in the bloodstream, where few collateral channels exist.

Main arteries supplying the brain, and circle of Willis

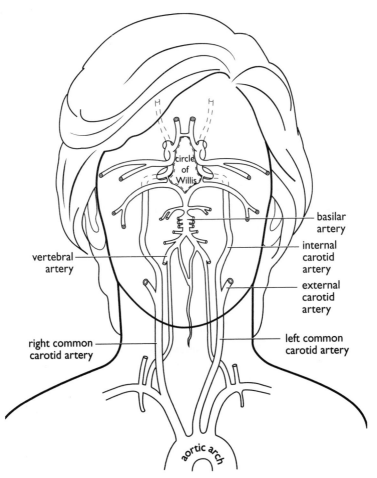

When the Blood Supply to the Brain Fails

When the blood supply to the carotid system is interrupted, the precise symptoms depend on where the trouble is. The carotid arteries supply all of the lobes of the brain except for the occipital lobes and the inner part of the temporal lobes. Usually, only one of the brain hemispheres is affected, and common symptoms are the sudden onset of weakness or numbness in the face, arm or leg. If the left hemisphere is involved, speech may be impaired. At times the only symptom of narrowing of the artery (*carotid disease*) is sudden, fleeting blindness in one eye (*amaurosis fugax*).

If blood is cut off in the vertebrobasilar system, there may be a change in the person's level of consciousness, because many of the functions that maintain alertness are centered there. If the cranial nerves, which allow us to feel and move our face and eyes, and to swallow and hear, are affected, there may be difficulties moving the eyes, double vision, difficulty swallowing, loss of sensation in the face or trouble moving the tongue. At the back of the brain stem are nerve pathways that bring sensation up to the brain; pathways at the front of the brain stem move the body, and in between are the vital centers that fill the brain stem. So it is possible to have a number of combinations of symptoms. There may

Blockages versus bleeding

There are two types of stroke: *ischemic* and *hemorrhagic*. Ischemic strokes (*cerebral infarcts*) happen when the blood supply to the brain is blocked, and hemorrhagic strokes happen when there is bleeding within the skull. Bleeding within the brain itself is called an *intracerebral hemorrhage*, while bleeding between the brain and the skull is called a *subarachnoid hemorrhage*. Eighty percent of strokes are ischemic and 20 percent are hemorrhagic. Hemorrhagic strokes are divided about equally between intracerebral and subarachnoid.

be loss of balance, double vision or impaired consciousness. If the cerebellum is affected, balance and coordination are impaired; if the back of the two hemispheres is struck, vision will suffer.

Because of the swelling and inflammation of the brain, at first it is hard to tell how much of the loss of function is directly due to the original injury and how much to temporary swelling, so the degree of recovery cannot be predicted with any certainty. In general, the sooner the stroke survivor begins to improve, the better the long-term prognosis.

Causes of Ischemic Strokes

Blood Clots
Blood clots are the most common cause of blockage of blood flow to the brain. There are many areas of the body where such clots can form. Not all blood clots cause strokes, of course, but if they dislodge and travel through the bloodstream to the brain, they do pose a risk of stroke.

The Heart
Atrial fibrillation is an irregularity of the heartbeat that occurs in 1 to 2 percent of the population and increases steeply with age. Blood can pool in the heart's left upper chamber and clots can form (see Chapter 3). One-third of all strokes in people 80 or older are associated with atrial fibrillation.

Malfunctioning heart valves also put people at a much higher risk of stroke. Valves may be misshapen from birth, or scarred as in rheumatic heart disease. Damaged heart valves can be the sites for clots or they can become infected.

Various other heart problems can lead to stroke. About 3 to 5 percent of people who have a heart attack will also have a stroke. After the heart attack, a clot can form on the heart muscle that has died, move into the circulation and end up in a brain artery. This cuts off the blood supply to part of the brain, causing death of brain tissue (cerebral infarct). People with diabetes and some elderly people can have painless heart attacks. Occasionally they have a stroke without realizing that they have also had a heart attack.

A whole-hearted recovery

Amy was an athletic 37-year-old. While skiing, she broke her left leg, which had to be put in a large cast. Then she developed a bad cold and spent several days in bed. One morning, she fell off the toilet and couldn't get up. She was taken to hospital and it was found that she had trouble speaking and moving her right side.

Amy had suffered a stroke. Being in bed had made her develop a clot in a vein of her left leg. But Amy had patent foramen ovale, a hole between the right and left upper chambers of her heart. When she strained on the toilet, the pressure in the right chamber of her heart rose above that of the left, pushing the clot through the hole and into the left side. The clot then traveled to her brain and closed off the middle cerebral artery.

The outlook appeared grim. Amy could only grunt. She could not move her right arm and her right leg was very weak. However, she began recovering within hours. Usually, the sooner recovery begins, the better the long-term outcome. And Amy was young and determined, and had an outgoing personality. Many friends came to provide encouragement and support. Amy's determination served her well through the grueling speech therapy, physiotherapy and other treatments, particularly in the early days when she had to walk with help on her weakened right leg, since her left leg was still in a cast.

After 9 days in hospital and 12 weeks of rehabilitation, some of it as an outpatient, Amy resumed her job as an illustrator. She could not type as fast with her right hand as before her stroke, and those who knew her well noted that when she was tired there was a hesitation in her speech and a slight limp in her walk. Aside from that, she was functioning normally. She had the hole in her heart patched, by a procedure done through tubes inserted into her blood vessels. A year after her stroke, she threw a party for her friends, including all the new ones she had met during her treatment.

A *patent foramen ovale* (oval hole) is a channel between the right and left sides of the heart, which is normal in the embryo and sometimes does not close up at birth as it should. People with patent foramen ovale are not usually aware of their condition. If a bedridden person with this condition has increased pressure in the right side of the heart from coughing or sneezing, a clot that has formed in the leg or pelvis can, rarely, travel directly from the right to the left side of the heart and up to the brain, causing a stroke.

The Arteries
Atherosclerosis of the carotid, vertebral and basilar arteries is the main cause of stroke.

Accidental damage to arteries can also cause stroke. Arteries have three layers. Sudden twists of the neck or direct injury to the neck arteries can cause the layers to shear from each other (*dissection*). This may cause the blood vessel itself to close, or it may cause a clot that closes the neck artery or travels to block a brain artery, causing a stroke.

The rupture of small arteries in the brain results in intra-cerebral hemorrhage, whereas blockage of the same vessels causes small deep areas of dead tissue (*lacunar infarcts*). This

---

Hardening of the arteries

As we age, small streaks of fat settle in the walls of the arteries. In fact, this can begin when we are in our twenties, in the main artery flowing out of the heart (*aorta*). These fatty streaks often grow into roughened, grooved *atherosclerotic plaques* that can trap cells from the blood (including *platelets*, the cells that start the clotting process). The plaques can become inflamed and crown themselves with clots. The term "athero-sclerosis" reflects the soft porridge-like core ("athero") and the harder fibrous tissue element ("sclerosis"). The plaques can crack and fester, breeding clots that can either close off an artery or be washed into the bloodstream. If the clots reach the brain, they can cause a stroke.

Ischemic and hemorrhagic stroke

arterial wall

blood
flow

Normal brain artery

atherosclerotic plaque

Artery narrowed by atherosclerosis

no blood
flow

blood clot

**Narrowed artery blocked by
blood clot (ischemic stroke)**

**Burst aneurysm
(hemorrhagic stroke)**

weak section of
artery wall
balloons and
bursts

is more likely to happen if high blood pressure has made the blood vessels thick, stiff and brittle. In people of African and Asian descent the main trouble often begins with the arteries within the skull, rather than those in the neck. These smaller blood vessels tend to undergo changes not only from high blood pressure but also from atherosclerosis and diabetes. Brain veins or venous sinuses (channels) can also clog from infection, or in rare cases from pregnancy.

Abnormalities of the Blood

Abnormalities in the blood sometimes increase the risk of clotting or bleeding, and occasionally both. Without enough platelets (clotting cells) people tend to bleed. With too many, their blood has a tendency to clot.

Too many red blood cells, a condition called *polycythemia*, can lead to blood clumps resulting in little strokes. Abnormal red cells, as in sickle cell disease, can collapse into sludge and close up small blood vessels; this is a leading cause of stroke among people of African descent.

In someone with leukemia, too many white blood cells are present, blocking the circulation in the narrower blood vessels, causing small areas of dead tissue and bleeding.

Clotting abnormalities can also lead to stroke, for many reasons. For example, *hyperhomocysteinemia* (see Chapter 10) results from abnormally high levels of homocysteine in the blood. Hyperhomocysteinemia has been associated with increased risk of stroke. It remains unclear whether reducing the levels of homocysteine decreases the risk.

Blood Flow Failure

Blood flow failure also causes stroke. For example, when someone suffers cardiac arrest (stopping of the heart), there may not be enough blood going to the brain. During surgical operations, blood pressure may be too low, with the same result. Blood flow can be thought of as water flow in a garden hose: if the pressure is reduced, the parts farthest from the hose will get the least water, or no water at all. This may result in damage in areas between the main arteries in the brain (*borderzone infarcts*).

Causes of Hemorrhagic Stroke

Bleeding into the Brain
The three main causes of bleeding into the brain (*intracerebral hemorrhage*) are high blood pressure, abnormal deposits in the brain's blood vessels in the elderly, and use of blood thinners (*anticoagulants*). Headache is common when someone has bleeding in the brain, consciousness is often affected, and the outlook is usually poor, because bleeding into the brain at high (arterial) pressure disrupts the brain's delicate structure.

Bleeding around the Brain
Bleeding around the brain (*subarachnoid hemorrhage*) usually results from bursting of a weakened outpouching or ballooning on a brain artery (*aneurysm*). An aneurysm develops on the wall of a blood vessel, usually someplace where the lining is less strong. Not all aneurysms are dangerous or require surgery; however, if an aneurysm ruptures, the bleeding is very serious.

Typically a bursting aneurysm begins with a sudden, severe headache, sometimes described as "a baseball bat hitting the back of the head." Other symptoms may include neck stiffness and double vision. About one-third of people who have a major subarachnoid hemorrhage have had a warning leak, a bleed that was not as severe. Indicators of possible risk are family history, a condition called polycystic kidneys, and smoking.

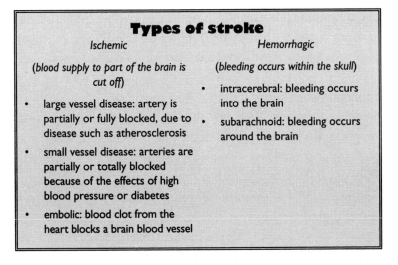

Types of stroke

Ischemic	*Hemorrhagic*
(*blood supply to part of the brain is cut off*)	(*bleeding occurs within the skull*)
• large vessel disease: artery is partially or fully blocked, due to disease such as atherosclerosis	• intracerebral: bleeding occurs into the brain
• small vessel disease: arteries are partially or totally blocked because of the effects of high blood pressure or diabetes	• subarachnoid: bleeding occurs around the brain
• embolic: blood clot from the heart blocks a brain blood vessel	

The second commonest cause of subarachnoid hemorrhage is the rupture of a cluster of abnormal blood vessels in the brain (*arteriovenous malformation*).

Mimics of Stroke

The shearing (tearing apart) of veins or arteries can lead to subdural or epidural hematomas (clots). The resulting problems are not considered to be strokes, but they resemble brain attacks and also require urgent attention.

Subdural Hematoma

Head injuries are the usual cause of subdural hematomas. An elderly person may bump his or her head and not think anything of it, but the bump may shift the brain and shear off some of the veins bridging the space between the brain and the skull. The dura is the tough membrane lining the skull. Blood accumulating between the dura and the brain leads to a subdural ("below the dura") hematoma or a blood clot. Since the veins have blood at low pressure, the blood oozes and may build up into a clot over a matter of days or weeks. Eventually the clot swells and puts pressure on the brain, causing symptoms similar to a brain attack. It may be difficult to identify the problem, because people tend to forget that they have bumped their heads.

Epidural Hematoma

Blood accumulating between the skull and the dura produces an epidural ("on top of the dura") hematoma. Sometimes, in cases of car accidents or other severe head injuries, a small artery that runs in the skull just above the ear (the *meningeal artery*) is severed. The blood spurts at arterial pressure, which is much higher than the pressure in a vein, and a clot builds up quickly, pressing on the brain. This is a medical emergency. The clot has to be removed very quickly to save the person's life.

Medical Conditions

Certain medical conditions can mimic brain attack, and need to be diagnosed by a doctor. They are:

- seizures
- a specific type of migraine headache
- certain infections of the brain
- drug overdose
- very low or very high blood glucose
- brain tumors

Heart Attack and Stroke Can Have Similar Causes

The most common cause of heart attack is hardening, or atherosclerosis, of the coronary (heart) arteries (*coronary artery disease*). The most common cause of brain attack (stroke) is also atherosclerosis, typically in the carotid or vertebral arteries. People who have a heart attack and people who have a brain attack often have the same risk factors for atherosclerosis, such

When a stroke is not a stroke

Despite being on holiday, a doctor was called to the home of an old friend, 88-year-old Arthur. A neighbor was worried about Arthur's behavior.

"What are you doing here?" Arthur asked. He was usually alert and articulate, but now he appeared confused and was slurring his speech. A quick examination revealed that he had a slight weakness on his right side.

"Arthur, we're going to the emergency department," the doctor said. Arthur's lifelong firmness hardened into outright stubbornness. He refused.

"If you don't come with me now, you'll end up in a coma tonight and you'll spoil my holiday," the doctor warned him, and Arthur gave in, not wanting to cause trouble for a friend.

At the emergency department, a CT scan revealed a huge subdural hematoma—an area of blood clots formed by oozing of blood from the veins of the brain. Much later, it emerged that Arthur had fallen in his bathtub two weeks before.

Arthur did remarkably well after surgery, and a year later he invited the doctor over for a drink, to celebrate, he said, "the first anniversary of the day you saved my life." The doctor accepted his thanks, but added that credit should also go to the hospital team, the conscientious neighbor and Arthur himself, who would not go to the emergency department for his own sake but did so for a friend.

as family history, high blood pressure (*hypertension*), diabetes, smoking, high cholesterol or hyperhomocysteinemia. But there are many more causes of stroke than of heart attacks.

Repeated bouts of chest pain, usually called angina, are a clear warning of future heart attack. If you have many warning signs, it does not necessarily mean that you are in greater danger. It means that you are at risk, but other factors affect that risk. The risk of stroke depends more on pre-existing conditions and risk factors than on how often the symptoms occur.

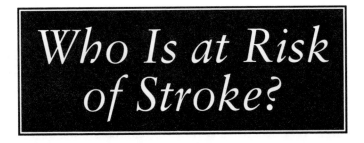

THREE

Who Is at Risk of Stroke?

Teenager, grandmother or toddler, you are never too young or too old to be at risk of stroke. The unfortunate reality is that there are causes for stroke at any age. Even an unborn baby can experience the harmful effects of a brain attack. Babies in the womb who develop hemorrhages or damaged brain from interrupted blood supply (*brain infarcts*) usually have impairments.

In children between the ages of 2 and 18 years, clots from abnormal heart valves and shearing of the layers of the neck arteries can cause stroke. In people between 18 and 45, the range of causes tends to be very broad (as opposed to the causes in older adults, which are usually more limited). Some of the more common causes of stroke in this younger age group are cardiac (heart) disease, shearing of arteries and blood clotting disorders.

Stroke in Adults under 45

Cardiac Disease
Some people are born with cardiac disease. Most commonly there is an inborn abnormality of the valves of the heart, or a hole between the right and left side of the heart that does not

close off at birth (patent foramen ovale—see Chapter 2), allowing blood clots that form in the leg or the pelvis to travel to the brain.

In a condition called *mitral valve prolapse*, the valve leaflets dip more deeply into the left ventricle of the heart than usual. This condition develops in the womb, occurs in about 6 percent of the population and usually has no serious health consequences. Very occasionally the place can be the site of formation of a small clot that is then displaced into the blood and ends up in the brain.

Shearing of Arteries (Arterial Dissection)

The shearing of an artery is another leading cause of stroke in children and adults. If a violent movement tears the artery, there are two ways the damaged artery may be closed off. One

A pain in the neck

Peter was thirteen and full of restless energy. He liked to play with older boys; he felt he was one of them. He chanced upon an improvised game of football and, uninvited, began to horse around. One of the older boys tackled him, put him into an arm lock, and, with a twisting motion, threw him to the ground. Peter felt a searing pain in the front right side of his neck. He picked himself up and began to run but stumbled and fell. He tried to get up but couldn't; his left side wouldn't move. He cried out. Michael, the boy who had tackled him, came over and noted Peter's scared look, and the slackened left side of his face, with drops of saliva sliding from the corner of his mouth. Now Michael was scared. He tried to pick Peter up, but Peter's left side was limp. "Stand up, stop fooling around," Michael pleaded, but Peter was not fooling around.

Finally a neighbor realized that something was wrong and called an ambulance. At the hospital it was recognized that Peter had suffered a brain attack involving the left side of his body because of the dissection of the layers of the right carotid artery, which had closed off the blood supply to parts of the right side of Peter's brain.

Peter was hospitalized and treated and made a good recovery, except for a slight limp, an awkward left hand and a crooked smile.

is that, if blood gets between the three artery layers, the inner two layers get pushed together, blocking the blood flow. The other is that, if the artery layers are damaged, they are no longer smooth, and there is a greater chance of clots forming on the roughened surface.

Any sudden twisting or trauma to the neck or head carries a small risk of brain attack. Car accidents and chiropractic manipulation can sometimes result in arterial dissection and stroke. Bungee-jumping, football, wrestling and boxing are examples of sports that may slightly increase the chance of this kind of damage. At times there is no apparent cause of the dissection, particularly in young adults.

Blood Clotting Disorders

A small number of people have abnormalities in their clotting mechanisms, usually because a protein deficiency makes them prone to clotting. A higher number of clots in the bloodstream increases the chance of stroke. Special blood tests are needed to identify those with blood clotting disorders.

Stroke in Older Adults (45 to 70)

After the age of 55, the chance of having a brain attack increases. The usual causes are atherosclerosis, cardiac disease and small vessel disease.

Atherosclerosis

The commonest cause of stroke in this age group results from narrowing and closing of the neck arteries that carry blood to the brain, due to accumulated deposits of fat inside the arteries.

Cardiac Disease

This is the peak age range at which heart attacks occur in men. The damage that the heart attack does to the surface of the heart muscle may favor clot formation, and clots may be dislodged and end up in the brain, causing a stroke. Weakened heart muscle can also bulge into a pocket (*ventricular aneurysm*) where clots are more likely to form, with similar results.

Atrial fibrillation (see below) is also an important cause of brain attack in this age group.

Small Vessel Disease

As explained in Chapter 2, when the smaller arteries of the brain become diseased, they can cause strokes. This happens most commonly among people with high blood pressure or diabetes, and in people of African and Asian descent.

Seventy Years and Up

The people at the highest risk of stroke are those over the age of 70. In the elderly, atherosclerosis remains the leading cause of brain attack, but heart disease becomes increasingly important.

Atrial Fibrillation

Atrial fibrillation (see also Chapter 2) occurs when the heart contracts irregularly, usually due to a blockage in the electrical pathways of the heart, which occurs with increasing frequency with advancing age.

Clots may build up in the left atrium—the upper left chamber of the heart—and be driven toward the brain by the irregular contractions of the fibrillating heart. A clot expelled by the heart and lodging in another organ is called an *embolus*, from the Greek "to throw."

Temporal Arteritis

Rarely, someone (usually over the age of 60) develops a painful, inflamed and enlarged artery in the temple. Aches and pains around the shoulders and hips may herald this. Temporal arteritis requires prompt attention because, unless it is treated with steroids, it can lead to loss of vision or a brain attack.

Amyloid Angiopathy

As people age, they are more likely to have deposits of a protein called *amyloid* in the brain's blood vessels. Amyloid angiopathy can occur alone or, particularly, in association with Alzheimer's disease.

The amyloid deposits weaken the blood vessels, making them more likely to rupture and bleed into the brain.

Finding the Cause of a Stroke, in the Old and the Young

Each age group offers special challenges in finding the cause of a stroke. In the young the number of possibilities is large and therefore requires extensive investigation. But even after a thorough investigation and tests, in about a quarter of these cases no definite cause will be found. The good news is that the outcome in this group of patients is often better than in those for whom a cause is found.

In the middle-aged and elderly, fewer but more obvious causes account for the majority of brain attacks. Sometimes there is more than one possible cause for the stroke. For example, someone may have a narrowed carotid artery and also an irregular heartbeat. Treatment depends on the causes. No test can absolutely ensure the right answer, but judgment and experience can usually determine the most likely cause, and the most promising treatment.

Strokes in the Very Young

Babies and even infants in the womb are at a small risk of stroke. Babies account for one-third of all strokes in the age group from newborn to 18 years.

Neonatology, the study of newborns, is a relatively new field of science, and many discoveries remain to be made. At present we have no way of predicting what children are at risk of stroke. Premature babies seem to have a higher risk and those who suffer a stroke as a child may be much more likely to have a stroke as an adult.

During the first month after birth, the baby is at the highest risk of stroke. This does not mean that the child has the same risk as a 65-year-old, but that the risk is higher than for a 12-year-old or 6-year-old. As you can imagine, it is difficult to diagnose stroke in a newborn. Diagnosis can be missed because the affected area of the brain is too small to be detected. Even if a CT scan is done, no signs may show up, because things can appear normal for 12 to 24 hours after a stroke. If a stroke is suspected, an MRI can be done to show the blood vessels and the brain, to see if a stroke has actually happened.

Newborn babies have no way of telling us about the symptoms of stroke, so it is up to an adult to observe the condition of the child. No definitive list exists of symptoms of stroke in children, but researchers have found that, in newborns, a seizure may be the first sign. (This is not true for adults. There is no evidence to suggest that an adult who has a seizure is at greater risk of stroke. In fact, the opposite appears to be the case; when an adult has had a stroke, the risk of a seizure increases.)

Researchers have found that most cases of stroke in newborns involve a blood clot blocking the blood flow to the brain. Systems that regulate blood flow and the clotting ability of the blood can be out of balance. Newborns in general have very thick blood because of a higher concentration of blood cells. If these cells sludge together, a blood clot can form and drift up to the brain.

In the first 48 hours after a baby is born, the circulation system goes through a change. For the past nine months the baby has been entirely dependent on the mother and now the system must adjust for the baby to function on its own. It is possible that, while the infant is undergoing these changes, a blood clot may form and go to the brain.

The leading cause of cerebral palsy is a stroke while the infant is still in the womb, which causes damage to the white matter of the brain, where the nerve fibers are located. We don't know exactly how the white matter is injured, or how to treat the damage. One of the times damage occurs is when the brain does not receive enough oxygen because its blood flow has been blocked or restricted (*hypoxia-ischemia*). The baby can be at risk at any time during the pregnancy, but particularly during premature birth. Initially, researchers thought there was a reduced amount of oxygen in the baby's system because the lungs were underdeveloped. They have now found that more organs than just the lungs are involved. Vital organs such as the heart and brain are still immature. The immature brain is especially sensitive to the reduced blood flow that can be caused by a blood clot.

Substance Abuse and Stroke

Drug abuse is a serious problem with many possible consequences. One is the increased risk of having a brain attack. Drugs such as cocaine, LSD, heroin and amphetamines are not the only ones to be wary of. Ecstasy, which has found favor with a younger crowd, can have the same devastating effect. Inhalant abuse can happen with over-the-counter medications such as phenylpropanolamine, or with various household products. Some younger children who do not have access to "street drugs" get their "high" by sniffing such things as glue, gas, freon, butane lighter fluid and hairspray. When abused, these household items can result in a devastating stroke.

Four uppers and a downer

Joe, a 25-year-old, took four capsules of street amphetamines ("uppers"). Within half an hour he experienced severe tremors, anxiety, palpitations (heart pounding) and profuse sweating. Fifteen minutes later he developed a blinding headache, lethargy and neck stiffness, and was unable to see the right side of his visual field. A CT scan showed bleeding into the front and back of the left side of his brain, and into the spaces between the brain and the skull, where cerebrospinal fluid circulates. Fortunately, the doctors were able to help him. After Joe gradually recovered, he signed himself into a rehabilitation program; no amount of "high" was worth such a terrifying and dangerous result.

Drugs can cause either a hemorrhagic or an ischemic stroke, in several ways. Hemorrhagic stroke (uncontrolled bleeding in or around the brain) results from ruptured arteries. Stimulants such as cocaine, ecstasy and amphetamines increase blood pressure dramatically. The sudden increases of blood pressure put a lot of stress on the blood vessels and over time can weaken them, making them more prone to rupture. If the blood vessels have a prior weakness such as an aneurysm or other abnormality, a rupture is much more likely to happen, and sooner. The higher the dose of the substance and the more frequently it is taken, the higher the chance of stroke.

Ischemic stroke (caused by blocking of the blood flow to the brain) can happen because of inflammation, infection, a clot or debris. Drugs such as heroin cause inflammation of the blood vessels. As a result, the blood vessels narrow and can eventually close off the passageway by which blood travels to the brain.

Illicit drugs that are injected directly into the bloodstream are much more likely to cause infection. If the blood becomes infected, there is a risk of clots forming and traveling to the brain. These clots can block off a smaller artery, leading to ischemic stroke.

Furthermore, injected street drugs may not be pure; they may have fillers to dilute the drug. Fillers can be as varied as arsenic, talcum powder, baking soda or cornstarch. After the drug is injected, particles from the fillers travel through the bloodstream and may eventually block off a small artery.

There is a long list of reasons not to use illicit drugs; possible stroke is one more.

FOUR

Women and Stroke

Typically, women think of heart disease and stroke as "male diseases," not likely to affect them directly. In fact, in North America, heart disease and brain attack kill more women than all other diseases combined. Not only does stroke strike more women than men, but it also proves deadlier to women.

The idea that stroke is not very common in women is the greatest myth about the disease, and women's awareness of stroke is far too low. Less than 10 percent of women in North America recognize the symptoms and risks of brain attack. Public education to increase their awareness could save many lives.

The highest risk of stroke is traded back and forth between men and women at various ages. Males are more likely to experience strokes before the age of 18. Between the ages of 18 and 45, women have a slightly higher risk of stroke than men. From the age of 45 to the age of 70, men are again more at risk. After the age of 70, the risk is about equal. But on average, women live longer than men. Since people generally have strokes later in life, this is one of the reasons more women than men suffer strokes.

Major causes of death for American women

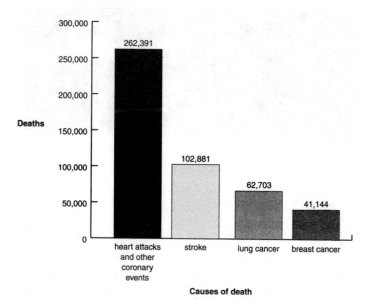

Statistics are from the American Heart Association and are for the year 1999

The onset of stroke is the same in both sexes. Immediate medical attention is necessary if you experience a sudden onset of one or more of the following symptoms: loss or slurring of speech; weakness or numbness of the face, arm or leg; double vision or loss of vision in one or both eyes; vertigo (a sensation of motion); difficulty with balance; an unusual, sudden or severe headache. Emergency care in the recognition of stroke has greatly improved over the years.

Some of the conditions related to stroke in women (for example, pregnancy and menopause) are directly connected with the reproductive system, and some are simply more common in women for unknown reasons (for example, migraine and autoimmune diseases). The incidence of stroke is increasing in women, as it is in men, but this probably has to do mainly with the aging of our society.

The Birth Control Pill

Oral contraceptives carry a slight increased risk of brain attack, especially in combination with migraine, smoking and high blood pressure (see Chapter 10).

Pregnancy

Women who are pregnant have a small risk of stroke, especially just before and after giving birth. During this time, changes occur in the blood clotting factors and a clot may travel to the brain.

Clotting in the brain's veins and venous channels (*venous thrombosis*) can occur with pregnancy or infection and put women at risk of stroke. Luckily, this is not very common.

Menopause

At the beginning of the twentieth century, the average woman began menopause at age 51, the same as now. However, the life expectancy from birth for a woman in the year 1900 was 59 years, and now it is 83 years. Not only will more women be reaching menopause, but more women will live many years after menopause.

Before menopause, women seem more protected than men against diseases such as heart attack and brain attack. Menopause seems to remove disease protection for women, making them more prone to these diseases.

Initial research into the effects of estrogen replacement therapy in menopausal women seemed to suggest that it reduced the risk of stroke and heart attack, but in fact the opposite is true. Taking hormone therapy, even for a short period of time, may put you at risk of blood clots, particularly if you smoke. The chance of suffering a stroke or heart disease increases slightly with the use of hormone treatment. The use of hormone replacement therapy for more than five years may be associated with a greater risk of breast cancer. In North America, seven women die from heart disease and brain attack for every woman who dies from breast cancer. Women should discuss issues of choice, side effects and individual risks with their family doctors.

Migraine

We don't know exactly why, but people who suffer from migraine have a slightly increased risk of stroke, particularly if they have classic migraine (migraine with visual symptoms).

Autoimmune Diseases

Women are more prone to illnesses in which the body attacks itself (*autoimmune diseases*). Among these are lupus erythematosus, which affects the skin and other organs. People with lupus often harbor a "lupus anticoagulant" in the blood. This factor, despite its name, tends to produce blood clotting and may lead to a stroke. Some women, and a few men, have the lupus anticoagulant without having lupus.

Bleeding around the Brain (Subarachnoid Hemorrhages)

Women are more likely than men to have a subarachnoid hemorrhage, which is usually due to a ruptured aneurysm. An aneurysm is a *bleb* (a small blister), most typically on one of the arteries at the base of the brain. The peak age for a ruptured aneurysm is 55 years, often at the height of life and productivity. If it's recognized in time, the bleeding aneurysm can often be clipped or coiled to prevent rebleeding.

How Necessary Is Gender-Specific Research?

We need to learn whether the protection that women enjoy until menopause can actually be extended to the postmenopausal period. Knowledge about treating women may also be useful in treating men. Understanding how estrogen works could lead to the development of chemicals that would give men the protective effect of estrogen without feminizing them—or perhaps identifying the protective properties of estrogen and not using the rest, since replacement of the whole estrogen molecule carries more risk than benefit.

Gender-specific research is important not only for women, but for all of us. The more we learn about a specific mechanism of disease, the more widely the knowledge can be applied. A number of special programs fund research related to women's health.

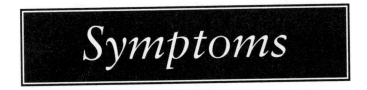

Symptoms

The most important way to protect yourself and others against the perils of stroke is to know the warning symptoms, particularly if you or one of your loved ones is at risk.

Take action if you have a sudden onset of one or more of the following symptoms:

- weakness or numbness of the face, arm or leg
- loss or slurring of speech
- loss or blurring of vision
- a sensation of motion (vertigo)
- difficulty with balance
- a sudden, unusual or severe headache

If you are experiencing symptoms of stroke, get help. *Do not wait!* Stroke is a medical emergency. The earlier you get medical attention, the greater the chance that something can be done that will make a difference.

What If the Symptoms Go Away?

Sometimes people have the symptoms of a stroke, but then the symptoms go away, usually within 15 minutes. Temporary symptoms can indicate a *transient ischemic attack*, or TIA.

TIAs are warning symptoms of impending stroke. They must not be ignored. People often think the symptoms are not serious and take no action, but if you have a TIA, you are at risk of stroke, and the fact that the symptoms go away does not mean the risk is over. You should be examined immediately. This is a medical emergency.

How Can I Tell a Stroke Headache from a Bad Migraine?

The symptoms of stroke are generally unusual and very sudden, developing within seconds. Sometimes the start of a migraine headache is confused with the onset of stroke, but it is important to remember that the onset of a migraine is more gradual. People often know when a migraine is coming; there may be visual symptoms or a feeling of nausea, and sometimes they "just know," from certain indescribable feelings. When a migraine begins, it moves in within minutes, not seconds.

What Should I Do If I'm at Risk of Stroke?

If you are at high risk of a stroke, be prepared for the possibility. Make sure that you and those close to you know the symptoms of stroke, and how to seek medical attention quickly. Some families develop a signal of tapping on the phone, or use hospital monitoring systems, in case they are unable to call for help on their own.

S I X

Diagnosis

The importance of identifying stroke as a medical emergency has been underrated in the past, partly because it was assumed that not much could be done for stroke patients. Today, the picture is changing. There is increased awareness of the dangers of stroke, and of the possibility of reducing the damage by taking quick, effective action.

The brain is thought to be mysterious and difficult to understand. The reality is that neurological emergencies are no more difficult to handle than any other emergencies, although the question of follow-up may be more complex.

What Happens in the Emergency Department?

When you go to the emergency department, the first person you meet may be a *triage* nurse who decides how serious the problem is. An emergency doctor will then assess your condition. Next, a neurologist, internist or family physician will be called to take over the continuing care. In smaller hospitals, family physicians may assess their own patients in the emergency department and look after them thereafter.

There are three steps in the assessment of a patient: the medical history, the examination and diagnostic tests.

> ## **What's a neurologist?**
> Neurology is the study of diseases of the nervous system. The nervous system consists of the brain, the spinal cord, the nerves and the muscles. A neuro*logist* is a medical specialist who mainly treats diseases of the nervous system that respond to medications. Neuro*surgeons* mainly treat diseases of the nervous system that can be corrected with surgery.

Assessing the Patient

The first step is getting your medical history. The doctor will ask for a description of your symptoms and how they first appeared. This is the most important stage of the assessment. You should also provide as much information as possible about earlier warning symptoms, your family history, problems in other parts of your body, medications you take, and your present state and any worries you have.

The second step in diagnosis is the physical examination. Your doctor may discover factors that are contributing to your symptoms, such as an irregular heartbeat, as well as assessing the severity and type of stroke symptoms you are experiencing, such as weakness on one side.

Testing the Brain

The third step in diagnosis is testing. Doctors will examine images of your brain, looking for several things. First, they need to determine if there is blood in the brain and, if so, where. They will look for early evidence of dead tissue in the part of the brain that has been deprived of blood. (In some cases the evidence of dead brain tissue will not show up for hours.) Finally, they will check for other possible causes of your symptoms—conditions that can mimic stroke, such as a growing brain tumor.

Two methods are used to obtain an image of the brain: *computerized tomography scan* and *magnetic resonance imaging*.

Computerized Tomography (CT) Scan

In this test, X-rays are beamed in such a way as to reveal the structure of the brain. Your head is placed in a device that looks like a big salon hair dryer. It's a painless procedure; all you have to do is lie back and relax while a picture is taken.

Magnetic Resonance Imaging (MRI)

Magnetic resonance imaging uses radio frequencies to displace water molecules slightly, after a portion of them have been aligned in a strong magnetic field. As the molecules regain their original positions they give off magnetic energy in the brain, which is captured in an image. With the MRI it is also possible to make pictures of the blood vessels in the head and neck. This process does not use any radiation.

MRI technology is advancing at a tremendous rate, and yielding more and more information. In places where it's available, it's becoming the imaging method of choice.

Testing Blood and Spinal Fluid

Ultrasonography

Ultrasonography measures the speed of the blood flow by the *Doppler principle*. When a train comes toward you, passes and then goes away, the sound changes because the sound waves are compressed. The speed and position of the train can be measured by analyzing the sounds. The same principle is used to calculate the speed of blood. Ultrasonography also produces a picture of the blood vessel.

Carotid Doppler

The *carotid Doppler* test is used to see whether there is a narrowing in the arteries of the neck. A device is moved up and down the neck until the artery is imaged and measurements of blood velocity are made. In most laboratories, an image of the blood vessel can also be produced.

Transcranial Doppler
The *transcranial Doppler* is an ultrasound technique that gives information about the blood flow in the main arteries of the brain.

Spinal Puncture, or Spinal Tap
In this procedure a small needle is put between the vertebrae in the back and a sample is taken of the cerebrospinal fluid, which normally bathes the brain and spinal cord. This test helps detect bleeding into the head. Spinal puncture is not used as much as it used to be, because brain imaging can usually detect the presence of blood. Occasionally it is used when bleeding around the brain is suspected but is not seen on the CT scan or MRI. If the blood is diluted in the cerebrospinal fluid it may not show up in the images, but it will be obvious when the fluid is analyzed. The procedure is uncomfortable, but a local anesthetic minimizes the discomfort.

Blood Tests
Various blood tests are done to identify problems that could complicate stroke treatment.

Hemoglobin
Oxygen is essential for the survival of brain cells. Hemoglobin, a protein found in red blood cells, carries the oxygen in the blood. A person with low hemoglobin (*anemia*) will have less oxygen carried to the brain. However, if there are too many red blood cells the hemoglobin level will be high and the blood will tend to be thick and "sludgy," and may cause little strokes.

White Cell Count
White blood cells fight infection. An unusually large quantity of them in the blood suggests the presence of an infection. If the white cell count is hugely elevated, it may mean that the person has leukemia, a cancer of the blood. If there are too few white blood cells (*leukopenia*), the bone marrow is not producing enough of these cells.

Bleeding Time and Prothrombin Time
These are measures of how long it takes blood to clot. They are used to calculate the dose of blood thinners needed.

Blood Sugar (Glucose)
Glucose is the only nutrient used by the brain. If the blood sugar is low (*hypoglycemia*), the brain will not have the energy to function. Hypoglycemia can also cause symptoms that mimic stroke. Too much blood glucose (*hyperglycemia*) is seen with diabetes.

Electrolytes
These essential elements in the blood include sodium, potassium and chloride. Electrolytes are important for fluid balance and organ function. Imbalances in electrolytes can cause weakness and irregularities of the heartbeat.

Testing the Heart
The *echocardiogram* and *electrocardiogram* (ECG) are used to search for any abnormality of the heart that could have caused the brain attack.

Echocardiogram
Ultrasound is beamed through the chest (*transthoracic echocardiogram*) or from a thin tube placed in the esophagus, the

passage connecting the mouth to the stomach (*transesophageal echocardiogram*), to create an image of the beating heart. The echocardiogram will show whether the walls of the heart are enlarged or damaged, and whether there are any pockets that may harbor clots. The echocardiogram will also show whether the valves of the heart are normal or abnormal. An abnormal heart valve may have clots or growths on it. Clots and tumors may also be found within the heart.

Electrocardiogram (ECG)

Several electrodes are placed on the chest to map the heartbeat. Problems that can be spotted by an electrocardiogram include irregular heartbeat (arrhythmia), an insufficient amount of blood being supplied to the heart (ischemia) or a part of the heart that has died because of inadequate blood supply (infarct).

Other Tests

Depending on the person's history, liver and kidney tests may also be done to detect damage.

Whatever tests are ordered, however, the most important part of the diagnosis is the doctor's judgment.

Treatment

lthough people who have had a stroke can be treated in a variety of settings, the ideal place is in a stroke unit, where the nurses, doctors and therapists make up a specialized team with the expertise to ensure that you get the very best care. In North America only a small minority of stroke patients are treated in stroke units. However, the number of stroke units is rising because of their obvious benefits.

It has been shown that if people are cared for by a team of experts in a stroke unit, their mortality rate is reduced by 22 percent, their hospital stay is shortened by 40 percent, and 16 percent more people go home instead of into a nursing home compared to those treated in regular hospital beds.

The overall medical treatment includes general and specific measures, and occasionally surgery.

General Measures
General measures are aimed at keeping the body functioning within a healthy range.

Maintaining Blood Pressure
The ability of the brain to control its own blood supply (*autoregulation*) can be lost with a stroke, so that the blood supply to the deprived area depends on the blood pressure. The body tries to compensate within seconds by increasing the

blood pressure so that more blood will flow there. About 80 percent of patients who have had a stroke have an increase in blood pressure that usually then decreases on its own, over seven to ten days, to the person's usual level. If the blood pressure drops, the medical staff can give medication, so that the blood pressure is maintained.

Reducing Elevated Temperature
Temperature increase harms the brain. Even a rise of one degree centigrade will double the risk of death or disability. Prompt treatment is essential.

Normalizing Blood Glucose
People who have high blood glucose at the time of a stroke are less likely to recover. Reducing blood glucose when the stroke first happens may be of benefit.

Specific Measures
Specific measures are used in an attempt to reopen closed blood vessels, protect the brain and prevent complications. Recently there have been several advances in reopening closed blood vessels with clot-busting drugs (*thrombolytics*). Clinical trials are being done to find drugs that protect the injured brain.

Reopening Closed Blood Vessels
A heart attack usually results from a clot closing off a coronary blood vessel. Giving a clot-busting (thrombolytic) drug will often reopen the blood vessel and prevent death of the part of the heart muscle supplied by that artery.

Two drugs commonly used for heart attacks are *streptokinase* and *tissue plasminogen activator* (*t-PA*). The sooner the drugs are given, the higher the likelihood is of reopening the closed artery and preventing a heart attack. **Time is life.**

The commonest cause of stroke is also closure of a blood vessel, but only t-PA is used. Studies suggest that the earlier t-PA is given during a brain attack, the more likely it is to reopen blood vessels and the less probable it is that t-PA will cause bleeding into the brain. **Time is brain.**

Tissue plasminogen activator has now been used for strokes, but it has to be administered within three hours of the onset of the stroke, and under very close supervision. Out of every 100 patients treated, 12 percent will have a better outcome; they will be normal or near normal, compared to a similar group not given t-PA. On the other hand, t-PA causes bleeding into the brain area

A Christmas miracle and a winter tragedy

One day in early December, a middle-aged woman suddenly had blurred vision. She assumed it was a symptom of migraine, since she regularly suffered migraine headaches. However, within two hours she was taken to the hospital by ambulance, and the doctors informed her husband that she was in a coma and was not going to live.

A decision about treatment had to be made quickly. The neurologist suggested trying t-PA, a new experimental drug at the time. Recovery was not guaranteed. But the results were dramatic: within hours, the woman came out of the coma and was able to recognize her family; the next day she was conscious and speaking. She improved quickly and before the month was out she was well enough to celebrate Christmas. The hospital staff called her their "Christmas Miracle." The woman has since made a complete recovery.

But another patient was treated with t-PA a few weeks later. This was a 59-year-old man who had suddenly developed right-sided paralysis and an inability to speak. He reached the hospital in the early evening, within three hours of his brain attack; the timing seemed right for t-PA therapy. After consulting the family, his doctors gave him t-PA in the hope of reversing a devastating stroke.

Hospital staff watched him closely for two hours, but their hope soon waned. He grew worse, and a CT scan of the brain showed that the drug had caused bleeding into the part of his brain deprived of blood and softened by swelling. All efforts to save him proved futile, and he died a few hours later.

softened by stroke in about 6 percent of those treated. So it is still a dangerous drug that cannot be used widely. But t-PA is just the first of many drugs being evaluated, and in future we may well have more effective drugs with fewer serious side effects. In the meantime, t-PA is given only in places where there are experts in diagnosing and treating brain attack. Such centers must have high-quality brain imaging offered 24 hours a day, with skilled people to interpret it. These centers should also be prepared to deal with the consequences of bleeding into the head.

Recently it has been shown that another clot-busting drug (pro-urokinase) improves the outcome, if it's injected into a closed brain artery within six hours of the stroke. This drug is promising but has not yet been approved for general use.

A substance called heparin occurs naturally in the body and prevents clots from forming. Although it has been shown to prevent the formation of further clots in the heart, legs and pelvis in bedridden patients, its role in stroke treatment remains unclear. All drugs currently used for blood thinning can also cause bleeding. The search is on for related drugs that prevent clotting but have fewer side effects than t-PA. Some such drugs are now being tested in clinical trials.

Protecting the Brain

About a dozen drugs that have been shown in the laboratory to protect the brain during the blood deprivation of a stroke are now being tested with patients.

Some of these drugs block chemicals that are normally vital for the brain's function; when part of the brain doesn't have enough blood flowing to it, these chemicals spill from the cells and harm the brain. Other drugs soak up harmful *free radicals* that are formed when the energy stores of the brain fail because of a lack of blood and oxygen. Yet other drugs and antibodies block the effects of white blood cells, which can release harmful substances that plug up the smaller blood vessels of the brain.

Enhancing the Repair of Brain Cells

We are learning more about how the brain repairs injury. We know now that nerve-growth factors normally help develop and maintain brain cells. Getting these substances into the brain may help it recover more quickly. Similarly, specially engineered cells may be injected into the brain to help it heal. These treatments are in the experimental stage.

Combined Treatment

The best treatment may be to give medications that open up the blood vessels, followed by a cocktail of drugs, including "brain protectors" that counter the different breakdown mechanisms that harm the brain, and brain repair enhancers that speed up the process of rebuilding. With so many new drugs being developed and tested, we can hope for great progress in the future.

Surgery

Surgery is not used in the acute phase of brain attacks unless a blood clot is pressing on the cerebellum, the vital part of the brain that controls balance and coordination. In that case the clot is removed, usually with good results. By contrast, removing a clot from within other parts of the brain has not been shown to be of benefit.

The type of stroke in which surgery is most often used is bleeding around the brain (*subarachnoid hemorrhage*). If an aneurysm has ruptured, the brain vessels can go into spasm (*vasospasm*) within three to five days, causing decreases in the brain's blood flow and further complications.

There are two approaches to dealing with a ruptured aneurysm: wait a few weeks for the vasospasm to disappear, and then operate, or operate early, before vasospasm has a chance to begin.

The only problem with operating early is that the complication rate is higher than in delayed surgery. However, because vasospasms can cause further damage, the overall risk is usually less with early surgery. Plugging aneurysms with platinum coils (*endovascular* treatment) is a new procedure for some aneurysms.

If an aneurysm has not bled, but has been found in the course of an MRI or cerebral angiogram done for another reason, and if the aneurysm is less than 10 mm (.4 inches) in diameter, the patient is usually just followed. There is no particular urgency if it has not bled, because it has probably been there for quite some time. If the aneurysm is 10 mm or greater the recommendation may be to operate on it, treat it with coils or use a combination of both.

Preventing Complications

When patients lie in bed for a long time, the lack of muscular activity allows blood to pool in their legs, making them prone to develop clots. The clots may lodge in their lungs (*pulmonary embolism*) and produce lung damage or even death. Bedridden patients are also liable to infections. When limbs are paralyzed, the tendons of the muscles shorten (in *contractures*), and any attempts to mobilize or move the patient can be very painful. For example, a painful shoulder can result from loss of muscle tone, because the weight of the upper arm-bone is no longer held by the muscles, so it pulls the bone out of the shoulder joint. Lying in one spot can also put pressure on the tissues and cut off blood supply, causing painful bedsores. The good news is that several of these conditions can be prevented.

Nurses and physiotherapists monitor the patients' progress carefully and change their position frequently; they also support and exercise the limbs and encourage deep breathing exercises. At first these are passive exercises—the therapists do them for the patients—but as soon as the patient is able to move independently, he or she must do so. It is essential that the patient make an effort, with the care providers' help. Recovery and prevention are hard work that only the patient can do.

Treating vs Not Treating

Sometimes the damage caused by stroke is so devastating that survival would be more grievous than death. In these cases, the family will be told early on how much damage has occurred, and will be given some idea of what they may expect if the patient survives.

Within the first few hours of the stroke, it will become fairly clear what the outlook is. In order to be sure, the doctor will take time to verify that there will be no recovery—that this is not an exceptional case. It is essential to let the family know when a loved one has had a devastating stroke, so that they can decide jointly, with the doctor, whether anything is to be done should the patient have a cardiac arrest (which is likely). A decision to resuscitate the patient may only make it much harder emotionally to discontinue the ventilator later. Luckily, the issue arises in only a minority of cases. Sometimes a person who has suffered a stroke also has a number of other illnesses, or has not regained his or her mental capacity. The family may feel that their loved one would not want to survive in such a disabled condition.

In many Canadian provinces and American states, legislation exists that protects people's rights to determine their own healthcare. A person of sound mind writes down what she or he wishes to have done or not done in the event of catastrophic illness. This legal document of wishes is called a *living will* or a *healthcare directive*.

Living Wills, Healthcare Directives and Advance Directives

A healthcare directive or living will is one way you can provide healthcare workers and your family information about what care you want and do not want, at a time when you can no longer speak for yourself. People have wills to determine what will be done with their money and possessions when they can no longer speak for themselves. A living will is similar in that it leaves clear instructions about how you want your personal health managed when you can no longer make the decision yourself.

The main components of a living will are the living will document itself, power of attorney for healthcare, and (optionally) documents with additional instructions. The living will specifies how you want to be treated or not treated under certain circumstances. A healthcare proxy or power of attorney for healthcare is a legal document naming someone close to you to act on your behalf, should you not be able to do so. If you choose to have both documents, the healthcare proxy names the person to make the decisions and your living will serves as a guide to ensure that your wishes are carried out. According to your instructions, the person you have chosen to make decisions regarding your healthcare can do so in one of two ways: using his or her own best judgment, or acting the way he or she believes you would act. That is why it is so important to have your wishes made clear to the loved ones closest to you.

Additional instructions are an important part of the living will. These allow you to be very detailed and specific about your wishes concerning your care. They may cover such matters as organ donation and what should happen if you become incapacitated while pregnant. Your choices and personal philosophy about medical treatment should be clearly stated in the documents. As with a will, you are able to change your healthcare directive at any time.

You are not obliged to discuss your living will with your doctor, but it is a good idea. The doctor can answer any questions you have, or explain treatments and procedures that you may not understand. Consult many sources to ensure that you think about many different scenarios. Think about how you would want to be treated if you were permanently handicapped, were in a coma, had suffered irreversible brain damage or were permanently unable to care for yourself.

Although the legalities of the healthcare directive differ from province to province and state to state, healthcare professionals are obliged to honor these wishes and do what is appropriate for you. In the recent past there has been much debate about healthcare matters such as euthanasia (mercy killing), but the living will does not and cannot ask the doctor to do anything illegal. At this time, euthanasia is illegal in Canada and the United States.

Your lawyer can help you construct a living will. You may also be able to obtain a living will by contacting the hospital, searching the Internet or, in the United States, accessing the U.S. Living Will Registry (see Further Resources, at the end of this book). If you are unable to register your living will online, make sure that it is included with your medical records.

Stroke happens suddenly. It comes as a shock. If there is no directive, and recovery is unlikely, the doctor will ask the family what the patient would have wanted done. Then the family is faced with making an extraordinarily difficult choice. The doctor's role is to explain the medical situation and give the family the support and time they need to come to a decision that is right for the patient and acceptable to the family.

If you make a healthcare directive, you free the family from the burden of not knowing what to do, or fearing that they will feel guilty about any decision they make. With a directive or living will, you are in control. Your wishes will be respected.

At any age, the time to consider writing your healthcare directive is *now*. You may also wish to consider the possibility of organ donation. Many people feel that this allows them, in a way, to live on. Is this something you would want to do? If so, include this wish in your living will, tell your family what you have decided and sign an organ donor card.

The decision to treat or not treat must be made by the doctor and family together, to make sure everyone involved gets accurate information. People don't always hear or remember accurately when they are under stress, and they may not understand what was said or intended. It's best if one family member is designated to communicate with the health team, to avoid inconsistencies and contradictions. This doesn't mean there will be no meetings with the rest of the family, but it makes communication clearer and simpler for everyone.

E I G H T

Rehabilitation

Strokes can inflict severe damage, but the brain has a remarkable capacity to renew and repair itself. Following the brain attack, unaffected blood vessels may take over the tasks of the damaged ones. If the problem was caused by a blood clot blocking the supply of blood, the body will try to dissolve the clot; medication can help with this. If the clot is dissolved before the affected part of the brain has been without blood for too long, the damaged part of the brain may be able to improve or even return to normal. While this kind of recovery occurs spontaneously with some people, most stroke survivors need an extensive rehabilitation program.

One of the most frightening aspects of a stroke is not knowing how it will affect you. The extent of mental and physical disability depends on the type of stroke experienced and where it has damaged the brain. Even subtle differences in behavior or the ability to perform tasks can be frustrating for both the survivor and the caregivers. The rehabilitation team helps the whole family adapt to physical problems, and counsels them on how to recognize and deal with the emotional effects of brain attack. Accepting that a stroke may have lasting effects is an important step toward recovery.

Accepting what you can't change

"I wouldn't have chosen to have a stroke and live the rest of my life as I am now, but it's what I've been dealt and I'm pleased with myself for making the best of it. While I don't want to idealize bad luck, we are more than our bodies and there's more than one way to fly."

Bonnie Sherr Klein, *Slow Dance*

The Rehabilitation Team

Stroke recovery calls upon the services of several health disciplines. Together with the survivor and the family, all these people work out the best plan for the individual. Key members of this team include the following.

The Stroke Survivor

This is the most important member of the team. Someone who has had a stroke needs to have hope, to try, to learn, to practice, to trust and inform staff and to decide to recover. The will to recover has a powerful impact on the degree of recovery.

The Physician

The physician diagnoses, treats and prevents problems arising from the stroke, and usually has rehabilitation expertise or training.

The Nurse

The rehabilitation nurse assesses plans and provides care for the survivor's physical and emotional needs. He or she administers treatment and helps the survivor and the family learn how to care for the person affected. Nursing assistants provide personal care, ensure bladder and bowel functioning and adequate fluid and food intake, prevent skin breakdown, and encourage balanced rest and activity. The nurse coordinates the care provided by the team and reinforces everything the therapists are doing. The nurse is the front-line team member between the survivor and the rest of the rehabilitation team.

The Physiotherapist

Physiotherapists help their patients keep the range of motion of their joints, regain strength and coordination and become as mobile as possible. They help people learn to transfer from a bed to a wheelchair and vice versa; then to walk, first between parallel bars, later with a cane; and at last, perhaps, to walk without any assistance.

The Occupational Therapist

Occupational therapists help their patients relearn the activities of daily living. Activities that are taken for granted before a stroke, such as grooming, dressing and feeding, may have to be completely relearned by the survivor. The ability to perform these basic tasks is crucial for someone who wants to return home.

The Speech Therapist

Someone whose stroke has damaged the left side of the brain may have a total or partial loss of speaking, understanding and writing. Speech therapists teach their patients how to communicate, and also look for difficulties with swallowing. A stroke may disrupt the coordination of the throat muscles and cause food or liquids to go down the windpipe, resulting in choking, pneumonia and occasionally even death. Difficulty swallowing can also lead to malnutrition, robbing the person of the energy required for rehabilitation activities.

The Dietitian

The dietitian recommends an appropriate diet with an individually tailored nutritional and caloric intake.

The Social Worker

Together with the patient and the family, the social worker develops a discharge plan and arranges for support systems outside the hospital, such as home care. He or she puts the patient and family in touch with survivor and caregiver support groups. Financial support can also be arranged when needed.

The Psychologist

Survivors often have a distinct change in behavior; some experience constant depression or extreme anxiety. A psychologist can help these people, and their families, by suggesting positive ways to cope.

The Role of Family and Friends

Having the support of family and friends can be very influential in the stroke survivor's recovery. Studies have shown that someone who has a partner tends to recover more quickly and extensively than someone who has no such support. Support means more than emotional encouragement; it means helping in practical ways, such as giving physical care, taking over home responsibilities or managing finances, without removing the survivor's sense of control, usefulness and dignity.

What Does Rehabilitation Do?

Modern-day rehabilitation is comprehensive in its scope. Its goal is to help the person reach his or her highest limit of potential recovery, in order to regain independence and return home. Emphasis is placed on teaching people how to manage their own lives in the face of change and possible disability. The healthcare providers support the survivor and his or her primary caregiver as they plan the required lifestyle changes.

Rehabilitation begins as soon as the diagnosis of stroke has been established and life-threatening problems are under control. The rehabilitation team works to prevent complications from the stroke, prevent a recurrence, mobilize the patient and try to assist him or her to resume self-care activities. It's important that the survivor be involved in all aspects of this care as soon as possible.

The immediate concern of the rehabilitation team is to prevent a second stroke and avoid complications that could lead to a delay in recovery. Precautions are taken to prevent, or recognize and immediately deal with, seizures and blood clots in the legs (*venous thrombosis*). If the person has swallowing problems (*dysphagia*) after the stroke, a feeding tube is inserted through the nose (a *nasogastric tube*) or directly into the stomach (a *gastrostomy tube*). This may have to be used until the person is able to swallow safely. Adequate nutrition and fluid are provided in a variety of other ways appropriate to the person's ability to eat and swallow. Medication and/or a catheter can maintain bladder and bowel functions. Sometimes, a seeming lack of bladder or bowel control is in fact an issue of speech. A stroke patient who is not able to communicate normally may have no way of letting medical staff know about a need to use the washroom. Fortunately, keen staff will pick up on this, and try to work out a communication system with the stroke survivor.

Avoiding bedsores and contractures by changing the person's position in bed is important in the early stages, and so is early mobilization. The physiotherapist performs range-of-motion exercises on the affected limbs, fingers and toes. The patient is not required to lift the limbs at this point; the physiotherapist gently bends and guides the affected parts through a normal progression of movement, called the range of motion, to keep the body limber. Gentle handling, progressive exercising and proper support of any paralyzed limbs prevent pain. The survivor's activity is increased as soon as possible.

Thinking Problems

A stroke may affect the survivor's capacity to think. It is normal to suffer a decreased attention span, a lack of concentration, limited memory, or decreased ability to make a decision or solve a problem. The person may have trouble remembering how to start a task, or be unable to carry out the steps required to finish it. Having simple step-by-step instructions will make it easier to complete the task, and practicing activities routinely will speed up learning. It is most important that the survivor slow down and not rush. Accepting that it now takes longer to think, make decisions or complete tasks will make the whole process less frustrating.

Emotional and Behavioral Changes

Stroke can turn a life upside down, so it is completely understandable that there are strong emotional reactions. Survivors

---

Recovery and relapse

Mary suffered weakness in the left side of her body, and was admitted to hospital. After initial testing and treatment, she underwent intensive rehabilitation. It seemed very successful, although she was not yet able to walk. Several days after she was sent home, though, her husband noticed that she was not carrying out the prescribed exercises, was not sleeping well and spent hours staring at the television set. This was very distressing to him, since it was so unlike the wife he knew. Moreover, whenever he tried to encourage her, she would melt into tears and complain that her life was over. After a couple of weeks of mutual misery, they went to see their family doctor, who recognized the symptoms of depression, explained that it was very common after a disabling stroke and prescribed medication. After a few weeks of treatment Mary began to sleep better, and her energy gradually returned. Eventually she became her old pleasant self again. She admitted that it had taken her some time to accept the reality of her stroke, and the fact that she would now have limitations. In time she learned to walk again, with the help of a cane or on the supporting arm of her husband.

A modern-day Christmas carol

"Mr. Scrooge" grew up during the Depression. He knew the value of a dollar—a 1933 dollar. Although he became wealthy, he was always saving for a rainy day and was frugal, even stingy, especially with his employees. He avoided doctors, but during an insurance examination he was found to have high blood pressure. He refused to have it treated.

Several years later, his family began noticing that his personality had changed. He would laugh heartily at mildly funny things and, more surprisingly, burst into tears when angry or moved. The real shock came at Christmas. In addition to the customary turkey for his employees, he handed out a generous cash bonus for everybody! One of his sons, who was involved in the business, spoke to the accountant and discovered that the boss had also made a number of rash business decisions. The family finally prevailed on him to see a neurologist, who established that his uncharacteristic behavior was due to a number of mini-strokes in the areas of the brain involved in emotion, personality and judgment.

may feel anger, frustration, anxiety, apathy or depression; all of these responses are normal. They may occur because of the brain injury itself, or because of the effects of living with the damage. It's important for stroke survivors to acknowledge and talk about these feelings, because it can help them learn to cope.

Emotional lability is a common response. It's the dramatic, uncontrollable swing of emotions from tears to laughter and back, often for no apparent reason. Knowing that this is common among stroke survivors, and that it will occur less often over time, may help the person feel less embarrassed, upset or worried.

But depression is the most common emotional response. It includes feelings of sadness, inadequacy and withdrawal. Depression is a natural reaction to any loss. When we lose a loved one, we grieve. Stroke survivors grieve the losses suffered as a result of their illness, and some become depressed. Patients with loss of speech (*aphasia*) are the most prone to depression. It's very difficult to go from being an independent individual to being dependent on others for even the most basic tasks. An inability to perform at the level of competence we are used to can leave feelings of anger, unworthiness and discouragement. Survivors sometimes feel so overwhelmed and powerless that they withdraw or lash out in anger. Psychologists and support groups may be able to help them come to terms with such feelings. Depression can usually be treated with medication.

Speech Problems

Speech is commonly affected when the stroke damage is in the left side of the brain. Speech disorders do not imply mental incompetence; they indicate that a part of the brain cannot function properly. There are two basic categories of speech disability, *aphasia* and *dysarthria.*

Aphasia is a disorder of language, both spoken and written. There are two main types—*expressive* and *receptive.* Expressive or *Broca's* aphasia is the inability to express thoughts verbally. This is by far the most common form of aphasia. People with Broca's aphasia are not deaf or incompetent, so shouting or talking to them as you would to a child is both insulting and inappropriate. They understand what people are saying to them and they know how they want to respond but they are unable to find and utter the proper words. Expressive aphasia is immensely frustrating for survivors and their families, and often leads to depression.

Receptive aphasia (*Wernicke's aphasia*) is the inability to understand spoken or written language. People can speak fluently but the speech does not make much sense. The extent of this aphasia varies, but it tends to be much less common.

Dysarthria is a disorder of speech in which words are slurred or hard to understand. The total voice quality of the individual may be changed, as well as the person's ability to control the volume of his or her own voice.

Speech therapy is usually moderately effective in helping a stroke survivor to recover normal speech.

Ignoring half the world

Nancy, a 72-year-old widow, did not respond to the knock at the door from her daughter Evelyn, who came by that morning to take her mother to the doctor. Evelyn used her key to enter the house and was startled to find her mother still in bed. She approached the bed from the left side and was surprised when Nancy asked, "Is that you, Evelyn?" but did not look at her, even when Evelyn was standing next to her. Evelyn called an ambulance. In the hospital it was determined that Nancy had suffered a stroke that involved the right back part of her brain (parietal lobe). As a result, Nancy ignored everything on her left side. When her paralyzed left hand was shown to her, she didn't recognize that it was hers. Food had to be placed well to the right of her before she would notice it. Nancy made a slow recovery, but not enough to safely live on her own.

Neglect of Body Parts and the Environment

When the right side of the brain is damaged, the survivor may be unable to see the left side of his environment. At times, this ignoring of the left side of the body and the environment is seen in someone who has no loss of vision on that side (*spatial neglect*).

Muscle and Movement Problems

Weakness

Following a stroke, people usually suffer some form of muscle weakness. This may be due to the muscles shrinking from lack of use, or because the muscle has been weakened by the direct effect of the stroke. The rehabilitation team works with the survivor as early as possible, to regain and maintain strength in the muscles.

Paralysis

Paralysis tends to involve one side of the body, so that the arm and leg on the same side are affected (*hemiplegia*). Generally the arm is more affected than the leg. Recovery tends to occur first in the muscles closer to the torso; in the shoulder and hip, for example, and only later in the hands and feet. Even if the leg fails to recover, it serves as a pillar (see "Spasticity," below) and can support walking. Hence, 85 percent of hemiplegics do regain some ability to walk, although it may be quite limited.

For those whose recovery is incomplete, walking may be limited to short distances in the house. These people may require a wheelchair or scooter bike to manage longer distances outside the home, such as going shopping.

Unfortunately, the arm is more of a problem. Fine hand movements are the last to recover, but without them that arm is little more than an assistant to the unaffected arm. Recovery of arm and hand function tends to be quite limited, and rarely reaches 100 percent. Much of rehabilitation focuses on achieving functional recovery of the paralyzed limbs, but if that proves impossible—particularly with the arm—the rehabilitation team teaches the patient one-arm techniques to help make up for the loss.

Spasticity

Spasticity is uncontrollable muscle tightness in the affected arm or leg. It is a common physical response to any injury to the brain. The brain loses control over the contraction of the muscle, leaving the muscle to contract independently and involuntarily. The muscle does not and cannot obey the nervous system's signals to relax, and remains in a stiff, taut and knotted position. In stroke patients, spasticity can be both harmful and helpful. It can result in painful tightness of joints, particularly in the shoulder and sometimes the hand; a painful shoulder is a common feature of paralysis on one side of the body. On the positive side, spasticity jams the knee and hip into extension (holds them straight) so they are hard to bend. Even if the leg is still paralyzed, spasticity will allow it to serve as a pillar, and with an ankle brace the patient will still be able to walk (although slowly and awkwardly).

If you want to identify with the stroke survivor, clench your hand in a very tight, strong fist. After a few seconds, it becomes difficult to hold your fist together with the same pressure; your muscles are tiring. After still more time, you will notice that it actually becomes painful to hold your hand in the tight fist. Now imagine the survivor, who has endured the ordeal of the attack itself and is now unable to control the tension or responses of the muscles in the body.

Spasticity may be reduced with recovery, but more often than not it remains. It is associated with muscle weakness and paralysis, especially in the arm. This can usually be identified by the arm being held close to the chest, with a bent elbow and wrist, and a tight fist. Spasticity in the leg can be identified by a stiff hip and knee, and a foot pointed down and in.

Spasticity should be suspected if you see the following:

- stiffening in fingers, arms and legs
- painful muscle spasms
- involuntary muscle contractions
- a muscle or muscle group that appears to be jerking
- abnormal posture for the individual
- hyperactive reflexes

Treatment for spasticity varies with the individual. Physiotherapists will move the spastic limb through a full range of motions to stretch the muscle. Temporary measures to help control the problem may include casts, splints or local anesthesia. Medication must be used with caution, lest it interfere with other medication being taken to control stroke. In any

The heat is on

Phyllis had had a long day. Since her stroke, she tired more easily, and when she was tired she was especially aware of the numbness in her left leg. "I'll just curl up on the couch and relax, and watch a bit of television," she thought.

She got settled with her heating pad on the left side of her leg and soon she was laughing at her favorite TV show. Before long, she dozed off. When she awoke, she realized to her horror that her heating pad had somehow overheated, and her left leg was blistered and burned. She went to the hospital, where they treated her burn.

"But why didn't I feel anything?" she asked the ER physician, who explained that, after people suffer a stroke, their sensation in the part involved is sometimes impaired. "It can be difficult to tell if something is too hot or too sharp, and you can really hurt yourself."

The physician suggested that Phyllis phone in a request to have someone check her home for her. "We can't make everything 100 percent safe, but many of our stroke survivors have had hospital staff or other care workers help them safety-proof things that were potential hazards."

Phyllis quickly agreed. "I want to stay in my home, and I really feel I can. But I don't want any more accidents like this."

"Well then, let's get you that phone number, and you can go on home," the doctor said.

case, medications for spasticity are often very sedating and only partially effective. In the most severe cases, surgery may be required, although this is rare. Surgery can help to straighten affected muscles where contractures have developed.

Loss of Sensation

Damage to one side of the brain can cause numbness and loss of sensation on the opposite side of the body. People with this problem must take safety precautions, or they may scald themselves with hot water, or suffer other kinds of injury, because they don't recognize the warning signal of pain.

Loss of Bladder and Bowel Control

Some stroke survivors have difficulty with bladder and bowel control. The most common problem is *frequency*, a condition in which people must empty their bladders more often, and must find a toilet quickly to avoid wetting themselves. Bowel incontinence is much rarer. Medications may help to reduce the frequency of urination, so that going out is more manageable and sleep is possible. Daily washing of the genital area and between the buttocks is necessary to prevent infection.

How Long Does It Take to Recover from a Stroke?

Neurological recovery tends to peak within the first few months and then taper off. In general, the earlier the recovery begins, the better the ultimate prognosis. Functional recovery—the return of the ability to do tasks—lags behind, but usually continues for a longer period.

Transition from Hospital to Home

Patient Assessment

Before someone is discharged from hospital, extensive assessments and plans for future care are completed. Clinical examinations review neurological deficits, medical problems and physical, cognitive, emotional and speech/language disabilities. The results, together with information about the person's living environment, family system and community support, are used to determine how the stroke survivor will reintegrate into the community. The opinions of survivors themselves, as well as their primary caregivers, are essential to any decision-making about their future care. Decisions about a suitable rehabilitation setting, attainable rehabilitation goals and (for someone who is unable to return home) the choice of community residence must be made in consultation with those most directly concerned. This is the time for the survivor and the family to voice their concerns and ask their questions, to

A poor recovery

Albert, a 78-year-old childless widower, was a diabetic with high blood pressure. He had suffered two heart attacks, and a stroke had left him with slurred speech and a clumsy right hand. One morning he woke up and found himself unable to get out of bed. When Sally, a retired nurse, came to the house for her routine check on him, Albert said he wanted to pee very badly, but when she asked him why he didn't go to the bathroom, he had no explanation. Sally found that Albert couldn't move his left side, yet he seemed strangely unaware that anything was wrong with that side of his body. She realized that Albert had suffered another stroke, this time in the right side of his brain. She called for an ambulance and Albert was admitted to hospital.

Because of his many health problems, Albert's outlook was not good. After five weeks in hospital and an unsuccessful attempt at rehabilitation, he was discharged to a chronic hospital. Although he recovered some strength in his left limbs, he continued to have difficulty knowing where his limbs were. His poor sense of orientation kept him in the chronic hospital for six months. Though he was eventually discharged, he continued to require nursing care in his home.

ensure that the best available care is selected for each stage of recovery.

Selection of a Rehabilitation Program

A variety of options are available for continued rehabilitation. People with unstable medical problems are usually best served by facilities that have 24-hour access to rehabilitation nurses and physicians, and to medical specialists such as neurologists. People who are medically stable but have moderate or severe disability are best served by intense hospital-based rehabilitation programs that can provide up to three or more hours of physically demanding rehabilitation a day. Lower-intensity programs that can be done at home, in an outpatient department or in a nursing home are ideal for people with minimum disability, or those who have completed the in-patient rehabilitation program. People in rehabilitation are constantly being reassessed, so they are not necessarily locked into a particular situation.

Long-term Follow-up

People who are able to go home will receive ongoing care in the hospital outpatient department. The outpatient rehabilitation team will generally follow them for up to a year; the length of time depends on how severe the stroke was and how well the person is managing at home. Those who have had a mild brain attack will probably be monitored for only a few months; their prognosis is usually quite good. Those who have had a moderate brain attack will be monitored for up to a year. For those who have had a severe brain attack but are still able to manage in the community, ongoing monitoring may be necessary.

A number of issues can arise once survivors are at home. They may have seizures, they may not be able to see a task through to completion or they may have difficulty adjusting to their losses. Having quick access to the outpatient department to get treatment and counseling often means the difference between managing successfully at home and being readmitted to hospital.

Preparation of the Home Environment

Before the survivor goes home, the occupational therapist will assess the home. Here are some of the questions that will be considered:

- Is the home accessible by wheelchair?
- Will the person be able to get in and out of bed without help?
- Will the person be able to function in the kitchen, and manage personal care in the bathroom?
- What safety features need to be added?

Arrangements for Community Services

Financial aid, home care, disability aids (such as walkers, or phones with larger buttons and handles modified for easier use), home equipment, meal delivery, housekeeping and local social organizations are some of the supports available in the community, all designed to help survivors function in their homes as independently as possible. The types and availability differ from province to province and state to state, and can usually be tailored to the individual's needs. Contact your local stroke association for guidance, or refer to the back of this book for useful resources.

N I N E

Living with the Aftereffects of Stroke

A stroke changes a person's life and sets new challenges. Advances in treatment, coupled with more sophisticated rehabilitation techniques, are now giving most survivors the hope of good recovery. Unfortunately, stroke damage often still leads to disability, difficulty walking or problems in managing daily tasks of self-care. The level of disability is influenced by the severity of brain damage, the medical treatment received, rehabilitation, therapies and the participation and cooperation of family, friends and the stroke survivor. The ultimate outcome largely depends on the survivor's attitude, determination and commitment to recovery. Even the most motivated patients may be left with significant disabilities, but determination can turn a life crisis into a different way of having a good quality of life.

No matter how small or great the disability, things will not be the same as they were before, for the survivor or the caregiver. The survivor's appearance or behavior may have changed. He or she may treat others unusually. There will be different stresses, additional responsibilities, possibly even a role reversal in the survivor-caregiver relationship. Needs and responsibilities will expand. Time will not.

The whole family, and friends as well, will need to try new ways of thinking, acting and interacting, to regain security in their daily life and relationships.

Physical Effects

Personal Hygiene

If you are just home from the hospital after having a stroke, you may find that maintaining hygiene is a challenge. Having an accessible bathroom and suitable bathroom accessories can make grooming easier. Ask to have all the products you use for daily grooming laid out in an orderly and accessible fashion. Liquid soap, soap on a rope or soap in a washcloth pouch may be easier to handle than a slippery soap bar. Hairbrushes, toothbrushes and bottles may be difficult to hold, but your caregiver can put spongy material around the base of these objects to

---

I eat right, I live right, why did I have a stroke?

Lucy, a 71-year-old professional woman, suddenly lost her ability to speak; the right side of her face slackened and she could not use her right arm or leg. Over the next several hours her condition improved, but she was left with a slight speech problem and awkwardness in the fingers of her right hand.

The neurological history, examination and tests showed that she had a severe narrowing of her left carotid artery, which was surgically removed, decreasing the chance of further strokes. She made an uneventful recovery.

Lucy was grateful that she had had only a slight stroke, but she was bewildered as to why she had had one at all. She watched her diet, exercised and drank only at celebrations. She had great difficulty accepting her doctor's explanation: living right does not guarantee that we will stay healthy and live forever. The wonder is not that Lucy eventually had health problems, but that she had been well for $2\frac{1}{2}$ billion heartbeats.

make your grip more secure, and you can test various brushes to see what's easiest to hold. Many products can be adapted for easier home use; be inventive. If you have trouble putting the cap back on the toothpaste, consider getting a toothpaste pump. If stick deodorant is too difficult, switch to a spray. Shaving may also be more difficult. An electric razor may be easier than a blade razor, or a man may prefer a trip to the barbershop.

If you are the caregiver of someone who is unable to manage personal hygiene, be prepared to help as much as you are asked to, but let the person do as much as possible. Sometimes this shift in the relationship—from being equal partners to being more like parent and child, for example—can put severe stress on the relationship. If this is a concern, consider getting someone else to help with daily grooming.

The stroke survivor should try not to wear pajamas or a hospital gown during the day, because they increase the feeling of being a helpless patient. If the usual clothes are too awkward, look for garments that are easy to put on and take off. Velcro-style closures in place of buttons or laces, and clothes that don't have to come off over the head, make getting dressed easier. Look for comfortable materials that won't irritate the skin, and remember that brightly colored clothing may improve everyone's mood.

Safety Precautions

Think about how you can avoid cuts and abrasions, particularly if there is a decrease in sensation in your limbs. Be careful about excessive heat and cold, too. Weakness or paralysis makes it easy for someone to fall, drop things or overlook injury to part of the body.

Cognitive Effects

Someone who is having difficulty concentrating, paying attention, making decisions or remembering is likely coping with the effects

Paradise lost, paradise regained

Arnold was a 67-year-old retired history professor with a near fanatical interest in old maps. Although he had enjoyed teaching, he had welcomed retirement so that he could devote himself to his maps—his idea of paradise. Apart from diabetes that required daily insulin injections, he had no major health problems.

One night Arnold appeared sweaty, pale and unwell, and complained of indigestion. His wife, Martha, could not convince him to see a doctor. The next morning he felt better but did not get dressed; he spent most of the day looking at his maps. The following afternoon, he was surprised that he couldn't orient his maps on the table. With growing frustration he kept trying to rearrange them, until his swearing brought his wife running. When she asked what the matter was, Arnold lapsed into garbled speech. This time, Martha put her foot down and they went to emergency.

Tests showed that Arnold had had a silent (painless) heart attack, a type more common in diabetics. This attack had damaged part of his heart; clots had formed on the damaged tissue and gone to the brain, closing off small vessels in one area that has to do with perception of space, and another that has to do with speech.

Arnold's speech recovered fairly quickly; the little clots blocking the blood vessels likely broke up, letting the blood through again. Arnold was put on warfarin to prevent further clots from forming. However, when he went home he found that he couldn't concentrate, and he had trouble reading some of the old writing on the maps. At times he could spell out the letters but still couldn't understand the word.

Arnold was dismayed by this, but he began devising tricks to identify places on the map, including little rules of his own invention. As the weeks went by, he needed fewer and fewer tricks. He continued to improve until, according to him, he had fully recovered. Had he? It's probable that he had suffered some mild damage, but his brain was able to reorganize itself to make up for his lost function—thanks to Arnold's great effort and desire to regain his paradise.

of the stroke. Both the survivor and the caregiver should be patient. Recovery takes time. Being slow in this area doesn't mean the person is stupid or incompetent, it just means that his or her brain is learning new patterns to retrieve learned information.

Emotional Effects

If someone's stroke results in paralysis or facial weakness, his or her body image will be changed. The person may feel no longer attractive, and therefore not worthy of attention and care. Maintaining personal appearance is one small way of helping people deal with this perceived change in who they are. Small luxuries that made them feel good about themselves before should be continued. A man who always dressed well and was careful to keep his hair neatly trimmed should be helped to maintain his well-groomed appearance; if a woman wore make-up, perfume and jewelry, she should continue to do so. If having a manicure and going to the hairdresser were satisfying activities before, they are even more important now, to rebuild body image. If such rituals were not part of the person's routine before the stroke, perhaps they should be introduced now, to bolster self-image and reduce the feeling of helplessness.

Many things can cause low self-esteem, but loss of independence and control is one of the most discouraging. To minimize this problem, try to involve the survivor in decisions, even small ones. Offer a choice; ask for an opinion.

Changes in Relationships

When a survivor rejoins his or her partner, various emotional issues may arise. Sexuality is one area where changes are often needed. Both partners may worry that the stress of sexual relations will precipitate another attack. Such fears are unfounded, but the physical functioning of the body may be different after the brain attack, and a doctor or sex therapist can address any problems. However, the new dynamics of the partnership may be more difficult to adjust to. For example, if impotence is a problem, it may be related to medications, but more often it occurs because the stroke survivor now sees himself as undesirable.

If the survivor is unable to manage personal grooming, and that responsibility falls to the caregiver, the very nature of the relationship has changed. It can be difficult for the caregiver to look at the survivor in a sexual way, yet the survivor may need sexual contact to support a sense of self-esteem. This very sensitive and complicated topic should be discussed frankly and honestly by the couple themselves. In addition, a doctor, couples counselor or sex therapist may be able to recommend ways to resolve issues, or to suggest sexual techniques that will compensate for the survivor's disability.

Self-help and support groups are available for stroke survivors. It's important to share your problems with other people who have had the same experience, and who understand your concerns. They may be able to offer a different perspective, or fresh solutions to your problems. They are also a reminder that you're not alone. This can be a great comfort, even an inspiration.

Care for the Caregiver

As mentioned earlier, when a stroke survivor regains independence, one of the contributing factors is often the support of family and friends. It's important for them to educate themselves about the aftereffects of brain attack, and to be patient and understanding during the long process of adjustment. Even though family members may agree to share the responsibility, it usually turns out, for practical reasons, that a primary caregiver (most often the spouse or an adult child) provides most of the care. This is a tall order, since the physical and emotional demands of the role can be overwhelming; he or she has a lot of adjusting to do as well.

The caregiver may be caught between wanting to show emotional strength, and feeling scared and uncertain. When someone who was always self-sufficient and outgoing becomes as dependent as a young child, or withdrawn and sad, it can be very difficult, even overwhelming, for the caregiver. Knowing that this person is relying on you for support can make it even harder.

Caregiver isolation and burnout can be a source of health problems. It is vital that you take care of your own needs as well as the survivor's. Set reasonable limits for yourself, and try not to do too much. There is no shame in asking for help. Many times, people would like to help but aren't sure what they can do. Divide up responsibilities for the survivor's needs, but make sure your own support system is also maintained. Work together with the survivor to find new ways to communicate. Plan something you can look forward to each day. Recognize that emotional outbursts are one of the aftereffects of stroke, and don't take them personally. The key to surviving your new responsibilities is to pace yourself, be flexible and keep a sense of humor.

Most important, don't hesitate to make your own needs a priority. For example, take a week off; engage in aerobic exercise; learn relaxation techniques; join a support group.

Acknowledge Your Own Feelings

Talk about your feelings, fears and needs with the healthcare team and your friends. Just knowing that they understand what the caregiving situation has done to you may help you feel that you are not alone. These are some common feelings:

Guilt

Don't let guilt rule you. Concentrate on the future, not the past. Be careful that you don't try to do too much, as a way of compensating for your guilty feeling. Make sure you can comfortably handle your new role. Caregivers frequently burn out because of loss of socialization and the often relentless needs of the stroke survivor. Take advantage of whatever breaks are offered, and accept help whenever it's available.

Fear

Fear can be the predominant emotion when you bring a stroke survivor back home. The most common fear is that another stroke may occur. That's always a possibility. However, if you are informed about measures that can be taken to reduce the risk, and you've learned what to do if another brain attack does occur, that fear can be minimized. You may also fear that you'll be unable to care for the survivor, or worry that he or she will end up in a nursing home. You may fear that the survivor will be unable to accept the new disabilities, or that your family and friends will abandon you. All of these fears are normal and reasonable; don't hesitate to talk to members of the rehabilitation team about your concerns, or to take advantage of the support systems available.

Depression

Depression is very common among caregivers. Focus on taking small steps, and talk to people. Things will gradually get better—if they don't, seek medical advice. A stroke is difficult for everyone involved, and it takes everyone time to adjust. Don't be hard on yourself; remember that you are only human.

Allow Yourself to Grieve

You need time to grieve for the person your spouse, sibling or parent once was. Coming to terms with this loss is an important step toward concentrating on building a new future. Remember that he or she *is* still the same person, even though it may take you a while to find the same qualities expressed in new ways, as well as other positive qualities you never knew your loved one had.

Prepare Yourself to Handle Emergency and Medical Problems

Ask the medical staff what problems may arise, and have them teach you any skills you may need to give medical treatments at home. You should also be aware of signs of complications, and know what to do. Call a doctor, or take the person to the emergency department, if any of the following appear:

- swelling or pain in a leg, arm or hand
- bleeding from the gums or blood in the urine, especially if blood thinners have been prescribed
- loss of consciousness
- shaking of one or more limbs
- pain
- weakness or numbness in previously normal parts of the body
- side effects from medication
- severe headache
- inappropriate or unusual behavior

Make Sure Legal and Financial Matters Are in Order
With this change in health, finances, wills and insurance need to be put in order if they are not already in hand. This may be an awkward time to deal with these issues but it will put your minds at ease for the future.

The Impact of Stroke on Family Members
Family roles and activities will most definitely be affected by a stroke, and the adjustments may cause tremendous stress. Changing the behavioral patterns and perceptions that have been in existence for a long time may be difficult.

What should a caregiver do?
- Ask questions of the medical staff.
- Discuss all decisions with the survivor and the family.
- Focus on the progress the survivor is making, instead of dwelling on what he or she used to be able to do.
- Know the symptoms of stroke, and what to do.
- Help with medical treatment.
- Don't shut out your own feelings; rather, acknowledge and accept them.
- Follow the guidelines for a healthy lifestyle, set out in Chapter 10.

While the family serves as the principal emotional and physical support system, social workers can be helpful in navigating the array of other support systems available to stroke survivors and their families. Not all strokes are disabling, and all survivors recover to some extent. As well, strokes can bring sudden awareness that we are all mortal and that we ought to make the best of the time we have left. Although it can be a catastrophe affecting the entire family, stroke will often bring a family together and also make members more health-conscious.

Support groups give survivors and their families and friends an opportunity to increase their knowledge about diagnostic and treatment options. Stroke support groups are generally set up for survivors by survivors. The interaction of the group helps to foster coping skills, and the meetings give all those involved a forum to express their thoughts and concerns, and to share their experiences of life after stroke.

Preparing Your Home

Before the stroke survivor returns, it's important to assess your home and determine what changes can be made so that day-to-day living will be easier for everyone. Since it may be overwhelming and costly to make extensive changes all at once, you may find it helpful to draw up a list of changes in order of urgency. Some survivors recover so well that house adaptations aren't required, but if they are, an occupational ther-

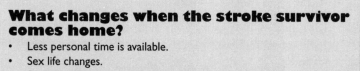

What changes when the stroke survivor comes home?
- Less personal time is available.
- Sex life changes.
- Survivors and loved ones may experience role reversal.
- All family members feel added responsibility and pressure.

apist can help you plan them. An occupational therapist may actually come to your home to recommend adaptations.

General Precautions

It's important to identify potential hazards. Should furniture be moved to make things more accessible? Can other obstacles be cleared away?

Do you have handrails on your staircases? Brain attack survivors often struggle with balance problems, and some are paralyzed on one side of the body. Handrails should be put on stairways, at a comfortable level, to offer reassurance, support and increased safety. Keep in mind which side the patient favors when you install the rail. If the survivor can't negotiate stairs, consider an electric lift. As the stroke patient improves, stairs that were previously daunting may become possible, so major home modifications such as an electric lift may not be necessary after all.

If the person is in a wheelchair, measure all doorways of the home. If it seems unlikely that a wheelchair will fit through the doorway, it is possible to purchase a device that will reduce the width of a wheelchair. The company that sells the wheelchair should be able to accommodate your request. Some people have trouble with door handles. If these are a problem, change the type of handle to one that is easier to manipulate—perhaps a lever—or remove the door altogether.

Stroke survivors will probably need more room to negotiate than they did before, whether they are in a wheelchair, using a walker or simply not as agile as they were. For this reason, it's important to provide plenty of space around tables, sofas and so on. Furniture that has sharp corners or may snag equipment ought to be moved to a more remote area. For someone who is in a wheelchair or has trouble bending, commonly used items can be placed on lower shelves or in other waist-level storage areas.

Flooring can also pose problems. Throw rugs have caused many slipping accidents. As a general principle, it's best to remove them unless they can be secured on all edges. Carpeting of the indoor/outdoor type, or with short pile, is safe. Carpeting with longer pile, such as shag carpet, is very difficult for someone with a cane, walker or wheelchair. Nonskid surfaces are ideal; if your floor is not of that type, avoid waxing it. Waxing creates an immediate danger zone.

Lighting is a consideration that is often overlooked. You need good illumination both inside and outside the house, so there's less chance of stumbling or missing a step. Nightlights in places like the bedroom, bathroom and stairways not only serve as guidance but can also make the dark seem less isolating. Make sure that light switches are easy to find and use.

Extension cords, cables and other wires should be tucked away as well as possible. It's best to run them along baseboards if you can, or attach them with electrical tape. As well as tripping people, loose cords increase the chance of breaking household objects.

Because stroke survivors are at risk of having another attack, and time is of the essence in an emergency situation, it's wise to have phones easily accessible to both the survivor and the caregiver. Place the phones in the rooms most frequently used, or consider a portable phone. Have emergency numbers close to hand. Since many survivors have impaired mobility, general safety issues become even more important. Make sure your home has all the standard safety equipment, including smoke detectors, fire extinguishers and carbon monoxide detectors. If you're not sure what you need, ask your local fire department to advise you.

The Bedroom

Consider putting the bedroom on the main level, particularly if the survivor has difficulty with stairs or is in a wheelchair.

A main-level bedroom may also be easier for the caregiver, who can carry on with daily tasks and still be close enough to respond to the survivor's immediate needs.

A lower bed may make the transfer from wheelchair to bed easier. It also lets the person swing his or her legs to touch the floor while sitting on the bed, to gain balance before standing. A chair placed beside the bed will provide added support. A lower bed also makes falling from the bed less hazardous. In some cases, a hospital bed may make care easier.

A portable toilet may be needed for a bedridden survivor or someone who needs frequent access to a toilet at night. A bedside table holding items such as a lamp, drinking water and tissues helps the person look after some of his or her own basic needs, but there should also be a bell for emergencies.

Bathroom

The first priority is to make sure that the bathroom is as close as possible to the area where the person spends the most time. Next, check the route to the bathroom and make sure any obstacles or hazards are removed.

The tiny space of a typical bathroom can be helpful to someone with balance difficulties, but a trial for a someone confined to a wheelchair. If possible, make space for the wheelchair to park alongside the toilet, tub and other facilities, to allow easy access.

Bars or railings in the bathroom are a good investment for everyone; we all know what it's like to slip on a wet tile floor. Bars installed beside the toilet and inside the shower or tub provide a good steadying base for a person whose legs are weak. Rubber matting or a nonskid surface can also help prevent a nasty accident.

A chair in the shower can make bathing easier, if the person can sit down to wash. Bath benches, which sit inside the bathtub, allow easy transfer into the tub and create a place to sit during the bath. A handheld showerhead allows easier manipulation of the water stream.

Large wing-type handles can be used on faucets in place of small tight ones. They are easy to turn on and off with a push of a hand or arm; a stroke survivor may lose balance and fall when trying to manipulate a small handle. A sink on a pedestal, without a cabinet, lets someone in a wheelchair get closer to the sink and mirror.

A high toilet seat may make the transfer to the toilet easier. Such seats can be purchased from a local supplier.

Make sure that all additions, such as bars, are secure and strong enough to support the individual's weight. Chairs should have grips on the bottom to prevent slipping.

Kitchen

Safety is especially important in the kitchen. Make sure the floor isn't too slippery, and wipe up spills immediately. Obviously the stove is a danger area. If possible, it should have burner controls in the lower front so it's not necessary to reach over hot elements. The stove is a danger to people with significant left neglect, as they may forget about items on the left side.

Taps are a particular concern if someone has lost sensation. He or she may not be able to feel when water is too hot, and may suffer burns. Hot water pipes should not be exposed. When running warm water, remember to turn on the cold tap first and then add the hot water as needed, so it's never any hotter than necessary.

People suffering from an attention disorder should not work in a kitchen, where they could forget an item on the stove. Kitchen assessments are routine in stroke rehabilitation. Working with the caregiver in the kitchen, as a team, gives the caregiver some help and provides the survivor with a way of contributing.

Adjusting the counter height and making cupboards more accessible are simple changes, and there are utensils and tricks that simplify work in the kitchen. For example, long-handled tongs make it easier to reach for items. Carts with wheels make storage easier and stored items more readily available; they can also serve as more accessible workspace. A cutting board with nails in it can make a world of difference to meal preparation. For instance, sticking a potato on the nails keeps the potato from slipping while it's being peeled.

Mealtime may be more time-consuming than it was before. Consider having one meal a day delivered from an outside source, or look for a healthy selection of prepared dishes at your local grocery store.

Recreation

Studies of survivors and their families have shown that one of the greatest difficulties following stroke is a lack of social activities and a failure to resume hobbies. Both the survivor and the caregiver need to be with other people, in the home and outside. If you are a stroke survivor, try, as far as you can, to

Charity begins at home

The Reverend Ralph was dedicated to his parish and his church. His three children were grown and had moved to distant parts of the country, and he hardly ever found time to see his grandchildren. His wife respected his devotion to the church and parish, but at times she wished he would give his own family the dedication he showed to others.

One evening he staggered into the kitchen complaining of double vision and slurred speech. His wife, who had coincidentally been watching a television show on stroke, surprised him by saying, "I'm calling an ambulance. You're going straight to the hospital."

At the hospital, he was indeed diagnosed with stroke. The family flocked to his side during his hospitalization. Realizing that all of them—including Ralph—had paid too little attention to each other, they made specific plans for regular visits. Ralph saw that he had come to feel he was immune to the very troubles he ministered to every day. After treatment and rehabilitation he was left with a slightly unsteady gait and occasional double vision, but he also had a renewed and much happier family life. Finally, charity began at home.

maintain the activities you did before. If many are now impossible, try to pick up new activities. Try to think of practical devices to make an awkward task easy. For example, a stand to hold playing cards allows a person with a disabled hand to participate more easily in a game. It's understandable that survivors often feel awkward with their new limitations, and that caregivers feel too tired to deal with the effort of leaving the home. In the long run, though, staying active and seeing people are important elements in recovery.

Transportation

Many people are unable to drive safely after a stroke. They may be easily distracted because of a lowered ability to concentrate; they may have impulsive behavior or slowed decision making. The most common reasons for no longer being able to drive are visual difficulties, left-sided neglect and partial paralysis. Difficulties with muscle weakness, or changes in judgment, or memory and perceptual problems may also influence the ability to drive. However, an inability to speak does not, and a card explaining this circumstance can be carried along with a valid driver's license. Problems that impair driving are usually detected during the rehabilitation process.

You must consult your doctor before attempting to drive after a stroke. The decision usually depends on a neurological examination, behavioral observations and an evaluation from the government agency that issues licenses. Where there is any doubt, a standardized driving test is recommended. Don't put yourself and others at risk by driving if you shouldn't.

If it's not safe to drive, there are alternative means of transportation available. Remember, getting out of the house will help combat feelings of loss of independence and isolation. Check the back of this book for further resources to help you find a service near you.

Handicapped parking spots are close to the entrances of public places, and they are also wider, to allow transfer to a wheelchair. To use this type of parking, you must have a permit. The permit may also allow you to park in some (but not all) prohibited areas. The permit entitles the driver or passenger (the person with the disability) to use these spots. You'll likely need a written statement from the doctor or physiotherapist. The social worker or occupational therapist should be able to help you get an application form from local transportation authorities.

If a paralyzed limb is the only significant aftereffect of your stroke, it's possible your car can be modified so you can drive. For example, an accelerator pedal may be placed on the left side, instead of the right.

There are adaptive driving classes for people who are deemed capable of continuing to drive. The final decision in each case rests with the agency distributing licenses. Find out what the requirements are, and ensure that you are prepared and equipped to drive safely.

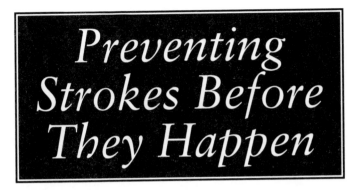

TEN

Preventing Strokes Before They Happen

Stroke prevention is infinitely more effective than treatment. By taking action to reduce your risk factors, you can significantly decrease your risk of stroke. But there are differences between *primary prevention* and *secondary prevention.*

Primary prevention includes precautions taken by people who have significant risk factors, but do not have symptoms. Secondary prevention refers to precautions that may prevent a second stroke in people who have already had a stroke (or ministrokes).

Assessing Your Risk

It is important to have a medical assessment to determine the extent of your risk, and what factors need to be modified and how. There are many risk factors for stroke, some treatable, some not. There are also some factors that protect against stroke. If you manage your risk factors and enhance your protective factors, your risk of brain attack will decrease.

Tables have been developed that identify different risk factors and indicate the probability of stroke in people who have some or all of the factors. The following questionnaire is based on the Framingham Heart Study, conducted in the state of Massachusetts.

How Old Are You?
Pick the one correct answer here, and add the corresponding points to your risk factor.

☐ Under 57 0
☐ Age 57 to 59 1
☐ Age 60 to 62 2
☐ Age 63 to 65 3
☐ Age 66 to 68 4
☐ Age 69 to 71 5
☐ Age 72 to 74 6
☐ Age 75 to 77 7
☐ Age 78 to 80 8
☐ Age 81 to 83 9
☐ Age 84 to 86 10   Score _____

What Is Your Systolic Blood Pressure?
Blood pressure is expressed in two numbers (e.g., 120/80). The systolic pressure is the larger number.

If You Are a Man
Pick the correct answer and add the corresponding points to your risk factor. If you are being treated for high blood pressure (hypertension), add *another* two points to your score.

☐ Under 105 0
☐ 106–116 1
☐ 117–126 2
☐ 127–137 3
☐ 138–148 4

☐ 149–159 5
☐ 160–170 6
☐ 171–181 7
☐ 182–191 8
☐ 192-202 9
☐ 203–213 10   **Score** _____

If You Are a Woman

Pick the correct answer from the left-hand column and add the points to your risk factor. If you are being treated for high blood pressure (hypertension), *also* add the corresponding points from the right-hand column to your score.

		with *treatment*
☐ Under 104 0	+6	
☐ 105–114 1	+5	
☐ 115–124 2	+5	
☐ 125–134 3	+4	
☐ 135–144 4	+3	
☐ 145–154 5	+3	
☐ 155–164 6	+2	
☐ 165–174 7	+1	
☐ 175–184 8	+1	
☐ 185–194 9	+0	
☐ 195–204 10	+0	**Score** _____

Do You Smoke?

If you are a smoker, add 3 points.   **Score** _____

Medical History

Men only: if you have a history of diabetes, add 2 points. If you have a history of heart or blood vessel disease, add 3 points. If you have atrial fibrillation, add 4 points. If you have an enlarged heart, add 6 points.   **Score** _____

Women only: if you have a history of diabetes, add 3 points. If you have a history of heart or blood vessel disease, add 2 points. If you have atrial fibrillation, add 6 points. If you have an enlarged heart, add 4 points.   **Score** _____

Adding Up the Score

You should now have four scores, for age, blood pressure, smoking and medical history. Add them up to get your risk factor. To determine your percentage risk of having a stroke over the next ten years, look up your risk factor in the appropriate table:

Men			
Points	*Risk*	*Points*	*Risk*
1	2.6%	16	22.4%
2	3.0%	17	25.5%
3	3.5%	18	29.0%
4	4.0%	19	32.9%
5	4.7%	20	37.1%
6	5.4%	21	41.7%
7	6.3%	22	46.6%
8	7.3%	23	51.8%
9	8.4%	24	57.3%
10	9.7%	25	62.8%
11	11.2%	26	68.4%
12	12.9%	27	73.8%
13	14.8%	28	79.0%
14	17.0%	29	83.7%
15	19.5%	30	87.9%

	Women		
Points	*Risk*	*Points*	*Risk*
1	1.1%	15	16.0%
2	1.3%	16	19.1%
3	1.6%	17	22.8%
4	2.0%	18	27.0%
5	2.4%	19	31.9%
6	2.9%	20	37.3%
7	3.5%	21	43.4%
8	4.3%	22	50.0%
9	5.2%	23	57.0%
10	6.3%	24	64.2%
11	7.6%	25	71.4%
12	9.2%	26	78.2%
13	11.1%	27	84.4%
14	13.3%		

Nontreatable Risk Factors

Age
In general, the older the person, the greater the risk of a stroke.

Sex
In the 45-to-70 age group, men have more strokes than women. Up to about 65 years of age, women are probably protected by the hormone estrogen, but within about a decade after menopause their risk becomes similar to that of men.

Family History
Family history is a definite factor, partly because a number of risk factors, such as high blood pressure and diabetes, are usually inherited. A family history not only of stroke but also

of heart disease suggests a tendency to hardening of the arteries, one of the most common causes of stroke.

Ethnicity

Stroke used to be the most common cause of death in Japan and in some of the major cities in China. Although cancer has now become the leading cause of death in Japan, stroke remains an important concern for Asian people. North Americans of African descent have more high blood pressure and more diabetes than a comparable Caucasian population, putting them at higher risk for stroke. The risk for Hispanics is less clear, since this group includes a wide range of ethnic backgrounds, including Caucasian, aboriginal and African elements. On balance, though, Hispanics are probably at a higher risk of stroke than Caucasians.

Personal History Risk Factors

Heart Disease

Previous heart attack is a risk factor because the damaged lining of the wall of the heart attracts the cells that stick together to stop bleeding (*platelets*), and a clot may form that can go up to the brain, resulting in a brain attack.

Strokes

Previous strokes put people at risk of more strokes, because they generally mean that the atherosclerosis is advanced.

Transient Ischemic Attacks (TIAs)

Not all TIAs result in stroke. The narrowing of an artery (*stenosis*), often because of an atherosclerotic plaque, causes little clots to form. These may go to the brain and cause temporary symptoms, and then break up with no further damage being caused. However, this is an indication that the person is at risk. Seek medical attention immediately.

Preventable and Treatable Risk Factors

High Blood Pressure (Hypertension)
The lower the blood pressure, the better, as far as brain attack prevention is concerned. With hypertension, the muscular walls of the blood vessels get thicker; if they didn't, the blood vessels would balloon or burst from the increased pressure. But there comes a point when the walls cannot thicken any more and they become brittle in the middle. This makes them prone to either closing off, producing a small area of dead brain tissue, or rupturing, causing bleeding.

High blood pressure is also a risk factor for heart disease. The heart has to pump harder, and therefore becomes larger but weaker. The combination of stiff, thick blood vessels and a weak heart is an almost certain predictor of future problems.

The good news is that high blood pressure can be treated and controlled. If you suffer from hypertension, you should take some precautions in addition to following the guidelines for healthy living. Seek your doctor's advice regarding medication to treat the condition, and severely limit the amount of salt (sodium) in your diet. An average healthy person should consume no more than 3 grams of salt daily. In our society, where convenience is key, many people exceed this daily recommended maximum simply by consuming fast food and prepared foods. Try to avoid adding salt to your food. Experiment with other flavorings to add zip to your meals, such as pepper, fresh herbs or citrus zest. Check nutrition labels to determine how much salt is in a serving, but note that labels can be tricky; watch for any ingredient with the word "sodium": sodium alginate, sodium benzoate, sodium bicarbonate (baking soda), monosodium glutamate (MSG), and so on.

You can also reduce high blood pressure by making lifestyle changes. Ask your doctor about these, or seek information from local health organizations.

Smoking

Smoking is a proven risk factor for heart disease and for stroke, both hemorrhagic and ischemic. It causes direct damage to the lining of the arteries (*endothelium*) by breaking down *elastin*, the fibrous protein that gives flexibility to the blood vessels. Since it does this to both the blood vessels of the brain and those of the heart, it also doubles the risk of sudden death from heart attack. Smoking is a particularly high risk for women. Statistically, men are heavier smokers than women, but women reportedly are more addicted to nicotine. The risk of a ruptured aneurysm in a female heavy smoker (35 cigarettes per day or more) is eleven times that of a woman of the same age who does not smoke. It is not known why this is so. Probably, smoking breaks down elastin, present in the skin and in the walls of blood vessels, resulting in wrinkled faces and weakened arteries. If you don't smoke that many cigarettes, are you safe from smoke's harm? Not likely. More research is being done on how cigarettes affect women, specifically on the impact of smoking on the blood vessels.

Hyperhomocysteinemia

In people with this inherited abnormality there are abnormal amounts of the natural amino acid *homocysteine* in the blood. Hyperhomocysteinemia is associated with early hardening of the arteries. If there is a history of heart attack or stroke in members of your family in their forties and fifties, you should have your blood checked. The good news is that hyperhomocysteinemia is treatable, although it is not yet known whether treatment reduces the risk.

High Blood Cholesterol

High levels of cholesterol (lipids) in the blood tend to be deposited in the lining of the blood vessels. High blood lipids, especially in combination with high blood pressure, get into the lining of blood vessels and build up abnormal deposits (*atherosclerosis*) that favor clot formation. These clots can break off and block a blood vessel downstream.

Diabetes

Diabetes is a risk factor not only for brain attack but also for small vessel disease, which occurs in the eyes, the kidneys and the nerves of the limbs. Good control of diabetes is essential.

There are two types of diabetes. Both types are serious health risks, not only for stroke but for other diseases as well. Both can be controlled but not cured.

Type 1 diabetes is a non-preventable disease in which the body has trouble producing insulin, which processes sugar in the body. The disease usually starts in childhood, and people with Type 1 diabetes must take daily insulin injections. Type 2 diabetes, which accounts for about 90 percent of all cases of diabetes, is largely preventable. Typically it begins in adulthood, but it is now being identified in children. Inactivity and unhealthy foods both contribute to the onset of the disease.

A nutritious diet, high in fiber, and an active lifestyle are the keys to preventing Type 2 diabetes. If you do develop the disease, these changes in lifestyle may delay the need for medication.

Note that diabetes can appear without warning symptoms. You may be at risk if you say yes to some of the following questions:

- Do any of your close family members have diabetes?
- Are you obese?
- Are you inactive?
- Do you have low HDL cholesterol or elevated triglycerides?
- Did you have diabetes during pregnancy?

Some people experience symptoms such as:

- unusual thirst
- extreme fatigue
- blurred vision
- tingling or numbness in the hands or feet
- frequent urination

If you think you are at risk, seek the advice of your family doctor.

High blood pressure, smoking, high blood cholesterol, homocystenemia and diabetes all damage the lining of the blood vessels. A combination of these factors increases the risk beyond the sum total of the individual risks—that is, the risks are not just added but multiplied.

Weight

It's not certain that obesity itself, in an otherwise healthy person, is a direct risk factor. However, if you are overweight you should consult a dietitian in order to start a weight-loss regimen of balanced eating and moderate exercise. A healthy body weight will improve your overall health and reduce your risk of other disorders that may lead to stroke, such as high blood pressure, abnormal blood cholesterol and diabetes.

The "beer-belly" type of obesity (also called the "apple" shape), in which excess weight is carried around the waist, is

---

Arterial diseases

Arteriosclerosis is disease of the arteries.

Atherosclerosis is disease of the larger arteries.

Arteriolosclerosis is disease of small arteries.

a higher risk factor than "pear-shape" obesity, in which the weight is mainly around the hips and thighs.

Chiropractic Treatment

Chiropractic treatment involving vigorous neck twisting can shear the lining of the arteries leading to the brain, resulting in a stroke.

Oral Contraceptives

The first oral contraceptives had a high estrogen content and were considered a small risk factor for stroke. The pills most often prescribed now have a lower level of estrogen. But the combination of oral contraceptives and smoking increases the chance of clotting. Smoking alone is a more powerful risk factor than contraceptives, but the two together create an even greater risk. Oral contraceptives also slightly increase the risk of stroke in women with migraine or high blood pressure.

Medications

Some medications (such as certain nasal sprays for congestion, colds and allergies) that contain an adrenaline-like drug will occasionally cause strokes. This is not usual or predictable, but is related to how often the medication is used.

A controversial diet drug, fen-phen (fenfluramine and phentermine), was taken off the market because it had been linked to heart valve damage, high blood pressure, seizures, heart attack, stroke and death. However, unregulated "herbal fen-phen" diet supplements remain on the market. The main ingredient of these supplements, *ephedra* or *ma huang*, is the same as that associated with the risks from fen-phen. Diet drugs in general have been known to be quite harmful. "Uppers," or amphetamines, used to be prescribed for dieters, but are now known to cause brain hemorrhage.

Substance Abuse

Cocaine can give rise to brain hemorrhages, and it increases blood pressure tremendously. This combination—weakened blood vessels and increased blood pressure—sets the stage for a major stroke. Heroin use also increases the risk of stroke dramatically, by causing the blood vessels to become inflamed. Moreover, the use of dirty needles can cause a blood infection in the heart valves which can produce clots that go to the brain. See Chapter 3 for more details.

Migraine Headaches

People who suffer migraines have a slightly higher risk of brain attack, especially if they have visual symptoms, have high blood pressure or are taking oral contraceptives.

Stress

Stress can be an indirect factor for brain attack. Most people with high blood pressure react to a stressful psychological test by having a modest increase in blood pressure. However, there is a group that reacts with great increases in blood pressure, and these people have a higher rate of development of atherosclerosis. The factor is probably not the stress itself, because no one can avoid stress, but how the person deals with it.

Protective Factors

Diet

A diet rich in potassium and fruits and vegetables is good for the heart and also for the blood vessels, helping to prevent stroke. A dietitian or family physician can recommend a diet appropriate for your age and weight.

One drink is equivalent to:
- 12 oz (or about 350 mL) of beer (5 percent alcohol)
- 5 oz (or about 150 mL) of wine (12 percent alcohol)
- 1.5 oz (or about 50 mL) of liquor (40 percent alcohol)

Alcohol

Moderation is the key. Growing evidence suggests that alcohol in moderation can act as a protective factor for both sexes. Some studies have shown a link between moderate alcohol consumption and higher levels of the "good" cholesterol, HDL. (A higher level of HDL is thought to protect against stroke because it makes the blood less likely to clot.) Wine is probably preferable to beer, and beer to hard liquor, but a modest effect has been noted for all types of alcohol. However, doctors are not necessarily advocating alcohol consumption. In fact, consistently having alcohol in high doses—more than five drinks per day, or binge drinking—is a risk factor for stroke, as well as heart failure, raised blood pressure and liver disease.

Women should limit themselves to one to two drinks per day, and men to two to three drinks per day. It is not recommended to exceed seven drinks a week and doctors advise against "saving up" your daily quota in order to drink a lot on one day.

Exercise and Active Living

There is probably not a single medical condition for which judicious exercise is not beneficial. It contributes to maintaining a healthy body weight, reducing high blood pressure and having a high level of "good" cholesterol, HDL. It combats anxiety and stress, and enhances a positive self-image. It also has a good effect on the heart and helps to prevent stroke. However, the amount and type of exercise must be suited to the individual. Your exercise program should be designed by a fitness expert.

How much exercise do you need? It's recommended that you be active for 20 to 30 minutes, at least three times a week. We used to think the 20 to 30 minutes should be continuous, but recent studies have found that the same benefits can be achieved by breaking down the activity into ten-minute segments throughout the day, which is more convenient for people who have trouble finding time in an already hectic schedule; they can complete a ten-minute segment of activity while (for example) waiting for a telephone call or listening to the news. As well, smaller segments are easier to accomplish if you are in a weakened condition because of stroke, or if you have never exercised and need to start slowly to build up your strength and endurance.

Does being physically active mean running and lifting weights? Not at all. The beauty of having an active lifestyle is that exercise comes in many shapes and forms. There is an activity suited to everyone. Walking, swimming and aerobics are very good activities for most people's overall health, but so are gardening, housework and dancing. Variety is important. Don't limit yourself to one activity; try several! Learn new skills and meet new people. Taking into consideration your ability to achieve and maintain a new activity, what would you most enjoy?

It's important to consult your physician before starting a more active lifestyle, especially if you are over 45 or have any existing health concerns, such as smoking, high blood pressure, high cholesterol levels, obesity, diabetes, a family history of heart disease, or residual effects from a stroke. Even if the doctor has given you the go-ahead, if you feel discomfort when you begin your exercise program, stop and consult your doctor right away.

Acetylsalicylic Acid (ASA)
An ASA pill a day reduces your chances of a heart attack. The dose can vary from 75 mg to 1,300 mg. (In the United States,

ASA is also called aspirin; in Canada Aspirin is a brand name.) It is still questionable whether it decreases the chance of stroke in people without symptoms, but if you have a strong family history of heart disease or stroke, aspirin may be beneficial. However, remember that this is a potent drug with significant side effects, such as gastrointestinal upset and bleeding; it should only be taken on a daily basis with medical advice.

Remember, living right does not guarantee that we will be healthy forever. With the best genes and a favorable environment, the human body may live for about 120 years, but eventually something gives way. A wise lifestyle and appropriate medical support can make life healthier and longer. Some day we may break through the 120-year barrier, but in the meantime it's well to remember William Boyd's words: "When all the natural frailties of our bodies are considered, it seems strange that a harp with so many strings should stay in tune so long."

What If I Believe I'm at Risk of Stroke?

If you think you may have a high risk of stroke, start by finding a family doctor with whom you're comfortable. Tell the doctor why you think you're at risk. Write a letter outlining your concerns, if that helps you to organize your thoughts. Then listen carefully to the doctor's responses. Do you feel this doctor can meet your needs? Do you have confidence in this doctor?

Unfortunately, not all doctors are knowledgeable about stroke. At the time when some of them were trained, there was no treatment available. Fortunately, stroke recognition and treatment have now progressed. The most important thing your doctor will do is identify the symptoms of stroke, and send you for a complete diagnosis and treatment. This can be a very difficult decision. The doctor has to be sensitive enough to detect real danger yet wise enough not to react unnecessarily. For each situation that is serious, there are hundreds that are not.

The doctor and you

You come to the doctor because you need help. Here are some ways to ensure that you make the most of the appointment.

Write it down. Some people get flustered at the doctor's office, and don't realize until later that they have forgotten to ask something. Write down what is bothering you, your symptoms, a list of medications you are on and any questions you have. You can also write down the advice the doctor gives you, so you have something to refer to after you go home.

Be honest. The doctor is not there to judge you. Topics that you may find embarrassing are topics the doctor probably deals with frequently. And don't omit information. Life changes such as a diet, new job or a new relationship can affect your health. You may not think there is a connection between your sleepless nights and your headaches, but the doctor needs all the facts to solve your problem.

Describe any treatments you have tried. Let your doctor know about any medications you are on, or have tried. This includes non-prescription drugs, especially herbal ones. As well, you may want to describe any health programs you are following so the doctor can observe how they are affecting your overall health.

Follow your doctor's advice. Once the doctor has decided on a treatment, be sure to follow the instructions carefully. If you are not clear about anything, ask for clarification. If you are taking medication, complete the treatment; for example, if you are to take the medication for a month, don't stop taking it after two weeks simply because you feel better. If, after a reasonable amount of time, the treatment is not working for you, schedule another appointment with your doctor. This is a team effort, after all.

You can educate yourself by reading books and articles and by obtaining information available from stroke associations (please refer to the end of the book for appropriate organizations). However, be careful not to fall into the trap of self-diagnosis. Know your family history, have regular checkups and, at the first symptom of stroke, get medical attention.

E L E V E N

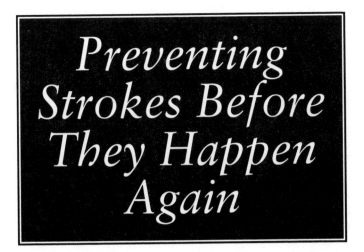

Preventing Strokes Before They Happen Again

Prevention is also effective after you've had a TIA or a stroke. This is called *secondary prevention*, and includes four main steps:

- Establish all your risk factors and treat or eliminate any that can be treated or eliminated (for example, stop smoking).
- Investigate the possibility of surgery.
- Use medication for any underlying physical problem that could lead to further strokes.
- Become knowledgeable about stroke.

Your Risk Profile
The first step, identifying your risk factors, has been dealt with in Chapter 10.

Preventable and treatable risk factors

- high blood pressure
- homocystenemia
- diabetes
- heart disease
- transient ischemic attacks
- oral contraceptives
- substance abuse

- smoking
- high blood cholesterol
- excess weight
- prior strokes
- chiropractic treatment
- medications
- migraine headaches

Protective factors

- diet
- exercise and active living

- alcohol in moderation

Surgery

The next step is to consider surgery. In the right patient, at the right center, with the right surgical team, the risk of a stroke can be reduced considerably by surgery. One of the most commonly and successfully performed procedures is *carotid endarterectomy*. This operation was first carried out in the 1950s, and it involves removing a narrowing in the carotid artery (in the neck) that causes TIAs or stroke. If someone is having TIAs, or has had a non-disabling stroke from a carotid narrowing of 50 to 99 percent, carotid endarterectomy can reduce the risk of stroke by about two-thirds. If the narrowing is less than 50 percent, or if it is more but not causing symptoms, surgery can only be recommended under special circumstances, which are best discussed with a stroke specialist.

Tests Prior to Surgery

Most of the diagnostic tests discussed in Chapter 3 are done after a TIA or a non-disabling stroke, but in addition, *cerebral angiography* is carried out. A thin tube (*catheter*) is placed in a blood vessel in the groin (*femoral artery*) under local anesthesia, and fed into the aorta, the body's main artery. The catheter is moved

On not seeing the light on the road

Paul, a 67-year-old, was driving home when suddenly a curtain seemed to come down on the vision of his right eye. He closed his left eye and noted that he had trouble seeing the traffic light with his right. That seemed to be the only problem, so he continued to drive. Three stop-lights later, his vision cleared. "That's funny," he thought, but he wasn't alarmed. But a week later the same thing happened again, this time while he was watching television with his wife. He twisted his head to continue watching. His wife asked, "What's wrong?"

"Nothing," he lied.

His wife knew him too well to accept this answer; she quickly got a confession about both episodes. With a little more effort she overcame his stubbornness and denial, and made an appointment with the family doctor. The doctor determined that Paul had had a TIA; he prescribed 325 mg of enteric-coated ASA a day, ordered an ultrasound of the carotid arteries and arranged for an appointment with a neurologist.

The carotid ultrasound showed 90 percent narrowing in the right carotid artery and 80 percent in the left. The neurologist explained that the ultrasound technique measures blood velocity and images the blood vessel, providing approximate dimensions for the narrowing. It does not show ulcers or vessels within the brain. A cerebral angiogram was done two weeks later, and indicated that a carotid endarterectomy was required. Paul was booked to be admitted for the procedure.

Under general anesthesia Paul's right carotid artery was opened and the narrowing was removed, in a three-hour operation. The surgery went well, and Paul was discharged with instructions to continue the ASA indefi-nitely, to decrease his chances of having a brain attack or heart attack.

up to the opening of the neck arteries so that a dye can be injected to show all four arteries leading to the brain.

Cerebral angiography is the only technique currently in use that can provide detail about the degree of narrowing in the carotid arteries, the presence of ulcers or a blood clot, and the state of other blood-flow channels that could compensate for a narrowed or closed artery (collateral circulation).

Angioplasty and Stenting

In this technique, a catheter introduced in the same way as for an angiogram is threaded up into the narrowed part (*stenosis*) of the artery. A small balloon at the end of the catheter is then inflated, forcing the artery open, and a metal mesh cylinder (*stent*) is placed in the expanded part of the artery to keep it open. This procedure has been very successful in the treatment of heart disease, and is beginning to be used in the neck arteries leading to the brain.

There are some unanswered questions about this procedure that may cause concern. There is a suspicion that clots may form on the stent when it's in place, creating a risk of stroke. There's also a possibility that atherosclerotic-coated plaques may be cracked or crushed open during the procedure, allowing debris to be washed into the brain, causing brain damage. Studies are being carried out to see whether angioplasty and stenting are as effective as carotid endarterectomy.

Treatment for Underlying Physical Problems

The third step is to treat any conditions causing the TIAs or strokes. In the two major causes, hardening of the arteries and heart attacks, clots can form and travel to the brain. Both problems are treated with two main types of anti-clot medication—*antiplatelet* drugs and *anticoagulant* drugs.

Antiplatelet Drugs

These medications block the clumping (clotting) of the small cells (*platelets*) of the blood. Clotting is a natural response to injury; if we cut ourselves, clotting stops the bleeding.

ASA

ASA (aspirin) was the first antiplatelet drug shown to prevent stroke. This opened the door to other studies demonstrating that aspirin also prevents heart attacks.

It is usual to begin stroke prevention treatment with ASA. One 325 mg tablet a day is the usual dose prescribed, but the dose may range from 75 mg to 1,300 mg per day.

Higher doses frequently produce side effects such as gastrointestinal upset and bruising. Serious bleeding may occur, but it is rare, even with the larger dose. However, for someone who can't tolerate ASA, or who continues to have symptoms, ticlopidine, clopidogrel or dipyridamole may be tried.

Clopidogrel
Clopidogrel acts on the platelets through a different pathway than ASA. Side effects include diarrhea and a skin rash, often transient. It is slightly better than one (325 mg) ASA a day, with fewer side effects, but it is more expensive.

Ticlopidine
Ticlopidine is a chemical relative of clopidogrel. It is better than ASA in stroke prevention, but because of rare serious side effects, including death, it has been largely replaced by clopidogrel.

Dipyridamole
This is another antiplatelet agent that may decrease the risk for brain attack, particularly in combination with ASA.

A common side effect of dipyridamole is headache, which tends to subside with continued use.

A patented combination of ASA and dipyridamole appeared in one study to be twice as good as ASA in stroke prevention, but the results are controversial. The combination is more expensive than ASA alone.

Anticoagulant Drugs
These medications "thin" the blood so that clotting is less likely.

Warfarin
Warfarin prevents clot formation in the heart, particularly in patients with atrial fibrillation and valvular heart disease, both of which predispose people to stroke. The dose is tailored to

the individual, to double or triple the time it takes for a clot to form. The coagulation of the blood has to be checked periodically for as long as the individual is taking warfarin.

The main side effect is bleeding. In any given year, about 5 percent of the people taking warfarin have minor bleeding and about 1 percent have serious bleeding.

What about Experimental Treatments?

Most university centers test experimental drugs and procedures that are not yet generally available. Most people who join one of these *clinical trials* find the experience a very positive one. This is especially true of cardiovascular trials, which have to do with blood vessels, heart disease and stroke. The participants usually have a better outcome than people with a similar condition who are outside the study, even if they are in the control group that gets a placebo (non-active substance) instead of the test drug. How can this be?

There are two probable reasons. First, everyone in the study is likely to get more effective treatment, because all participants are extremely carefully monitored and get optimal care. Secondly, once people have made a commitment to follow a treatment, they usually deliver on it. If people have been told to stop smoking, or to take pills on a strict schedule, they are much more likely to follow the advice faithfully if someone is going to ask them about their compliance and be keenly interested in their answer.

In addition to whatever benefits you gain, the knowledge you acquire may be useful to other members of your family. Another important reason that often motivates people to join a study, even when it requires a great deal of dedication, is the fact that they may help not only themselves but others with similar problems.

Typically there is an initial assessment of study participants, and then a series of appointments, usually months apart. Some studies don't require a long follow-up; those investigating acute stroke treatment are usually limited to an initial assessment and one follow-up appointment. If the trial is about prevention, however, participants may be asked to come for as many as five annual appointments.

Alternative Therapies

Before you consider non-conventional therapies, be sure you know what your problem is. *Do not self-diagnose*, especially if you have some medical knowledge. It has been said that a doctor who treats himself has a fool for a patient. It is important to consult sources and do your own research, but too often people diagnose themselves and decide on their own treatments. More often than not, they base their decisions on what they have read or heard from a friend. The first thing you should do is see a doctor and get a medical diagnosis. Then follow the treatment plan as outlined by your doctor. If after a certain amount of time you are still not happy with the results, and you want to consider alternative or complementary medicine, there are a few things you should do.

Find a qualified alternative medicine practitioner. Do as much investigation about the therapy as you can so you are informed when you are looking for a qualified practitioner. Then make sure the practitioner has any credentials and licenses required in your province or state. The first visit to the practitioner should be just a consultation, not an appointment for treatment. Come prepared with a list of questions to ask. There are guidelines available for the type of questions to ask, but some to consider would be: *Does your therapy help people with my condition? Do you have any evidence of this? Can I talk to any former patients? How much will this therapy cost and how many visits will it take before we can tell if it is working?* And the biggest question of all: *Are you willing to discuss your alternative therapy plan with my doctor?*

Discuss the alternative therapy plan with your doctor. After your initial visit with the alternative medicine practitioner, bring your research and the proposed plan of treatment to your doctor. This is an essential step, because you want to make sure the therapy will not interfere with your conventional treatment. This is also a good time for your doctor to voice any concerns, or comment on what is reasonable or unreasonable to expect from the treatment. Have your doctor explain his or her objections. Are they based on fact or opinion? Oftentimes alternative medicine can be complementary to conventional medicine, but sometimes it can be dangerous. It is crucial to keep your doctor informed about any complementary treatment you receive, whether it be acupuncture or a herbal remedy you bought at the health store.

Do not combine treatments. It can be dangerous to mix certain alternative treatments with conventional ones, and it can also be dangerous to combine two or more alternative remedies. When we are sick, we will try almost anything to get better, and fast, believing the claims and promises of anyone who offers a cure. It can be especially risky to try several complementary treatments at the same time because many have not been scientifically tested. If you are thinking of trying more than one therapy, prioritize the types of treatment you would like to try, based on research and your doctor's advice. Evaluate each treatment thoroughly in turn. Give each time to be effective. Do not evaluate therapies in combination unless your doctor thinks the combination is safe.

Plot your progress. It is a good idea to record how you are affected when you begin a new treatment. Ask your doctor if there are any objective tests, like measuring blood pressure, that you can do before you begin treatment. If not, keep a symptoms journal instead. Before you begin treatment, write down what symptoms you have and how you feel on a daily basis. Continue with the journal once you start treatment, writing down how you feel every day and what symptoms you have. After one or two months, review your journal and assess whether this treatment is working well enough for you. This can be a good indicator of whether the product is helping or just wasting your money.

Some Common Complementary Therapies

Acupuncture and Acupressure

According to anecdotal and scientific evidence, acupuncture may relieve pain. The ancient Chinese treatment involves the insertion of very thin needles into specific points in the skin with the purpose of regulating "energy flow" and reducing pain. It seems to help some people deal with the pain that can be a complication of stroke. A similar practice to acupuncture is acupressure, where manual pressure replaces the needles.

Aromatherapy

Aromatherapy uses oils—referred to as essential oils—extracted from plants to relieve health problems. Scientifically, not much is known about the actual effects, if any, of these essential oils. This treatment is based on diverse cultures' historical use of plants. The essential oils are used in one of two ways: inhaled through the nose or applied directly to the skin; they are never swallowed. Some claims made about aromatherapy are that it promotes relaxation, soothes muscle aches, enhances memory and eases pain. The best effect of aromatherapy may be that it relaxes the patient, thereby making the body more receptive to treatment.

Before using aromatherapy products, consult a doctor, particularly if you suffer from allergies, lung conditions or sensitive skin. Research possible side effects and note that the same essential oil can appear in varied concentrations in different brands.

Ayurvedic Medicine

Ayurveda was established over five thousand years ago, in India. It focuses on preventing illness and maintaining good health through balancing mind, body and spirit. It is thought that balance equals order and imbalance equals disorder, and that health therefore equals order and disease equals disorder, and that, if one can determine what has caused the disorder, things can be brought back into equilibrium. Order, or good health, is said to result from balance in life through lifestyle changes such as positive thinking, healthy diet, yoga, meditation, massage and herbal remedies.

Chelation Therapy

The American writer H.L. Mencken wrote, "There is always an easy solution for every human problem: neat, plausible and wrong." One example is chelation therapy, which consists of the infusion of a compound that takes calcium and other chemicals from the blood. Atherosclerosis roughens and clogs arteries, hardening their walls with deposits that include calcium. Some people claim that chelation therapy will leach out the calcium and dissolve the deposits, rendering the blood vessels healthy again. The idea of an organic Drāno unplugging the body's plumbing has intuitive appeal; why spend money and time on expensive medications, doctors and even surgery if you can have your blood vessels cleaned as easily as you can change your car's oil? Regrettably, chelation therapy is ineffective and even dangerous, because it tends to remove essential elements, including calcium, from the blood; this can make the person weak and ill, since calcium is needed for normal muscle and heart function.

Chiropractic

Chiropractic care claims to realign the body and reduce pain and other symptoms through manual manipulation. This is achieved by adjustments to the spine, which return the vertebrae to their natural state.

Chiropractic treatment can be a risk factor for stroke if a neck manipulation is performed. With a sudden twisting motion to the neck, shearing of the artery can sometimes occur, along with the possibility of stroke. This type of alternative medicine is best practiced with caution.

Herbal Medicine

Herbal medicine is arguably the most popular form of alternative medicine worldwide. Thousands of plant varieties populate this earth and many have been used medicinally for centuries. Herbal remedies are sold in a wide range of forms such as raw herbs, herbal extracts, capsules, tablets, lozenges, ointments and herbal compounds.

Instead of relying on the power of one ingredient, as modern-day pharmacologists tend to do, herbalists focus on the healing properties of the whole plant and how plants interact together. Since many herbs have not yet been studied scientifically, it is important to note the quantity of the herb used in each medication, and to educate yourself about potential side effects. Herbs are like prescription medication in that they can be very potent and should be taken with a doctor's supervision.

Hydrotherapy

Hydrotherapy is meant to improve circulation in the body by alternating the use of hot and cold water. Many of us already use a simple variation of this treatment when we use an icepack to reduce swelling or a hot compress for a headache. Usually, the patient reclines with the chest covered with hot blankets, and is then wrapped in a single sheet and covered with blankets. Once the patient has warmed up, one of the hot towels is replaced with a cold one. The body reacts to this sudden change in temperature by increasing the blood flow to the area where the cold towel was placed. This improved circulation of the body's blood is supposed to reduce pain and contribute to general wellbeing.

Massage Therapy

Massage is claimed to benefit all people, young and old alike. The rhythmic pressure placed on the body's muscles relaxes the person and can enhance flexibility. Some manual techniques of massage include kneading, stroking, friction and pressure. Most massages are even further enhanced by the use of oils, lotions and a relaxing environment.

Naturopathy

Naturopathic medicine claims that the body is able to heal itself. The approach is to seek out and treat the cause of the ailment, rather than the symptoms of the ailment. Lifestyle counseling is an important part of the naturopath's prescription for healing, as are a number of treatments already discussed, such as acupuncture, herbal medicine, hydrotherapy and massage.

Reflexology

Reflexology is a general treatment for the whole body. It does not target specific symptoms but rather works to bring the body back in tune with itself. Using their hands, reflexologists apply gentle pressure to the feet. The focus for each patient is different. The reflexologist claims to find imbalances in the feet that, when pressed, relieve tension throughout the whole body.

If It Sounds Too Good to be True ...

Some schools of alternative medicine advocate a good diet and a healthy lifestyle, encouraging people to take responsibility for their own health. These are all worthy goals. However, when extraordinary claims are made on no sound foundation—claims that may prevent the individual from seeking truly effective treatments—some caution is due. People have to realize that the claims of alternative medicine far exceed the proofs, and among the many true believers there are also unscrupulous merchants of hope, willing to prey on the credulity of the vulnerable. To safeguard against false claims, heed the old saying that if something sounds too good to be true, it probably is. If a suggested remedy is questionable, go to a respectable organization and get advice on it. If there is no solid evidence for it—if claims are made in the form of anecdote or advertisement—be very careful. Chances are that it is ineffective or harmful, or both.

Medical institutions are starting to set up programs to evaluate alternative medicine. This is a great stride forward in sorting the ineffective or harmful from the truly helpful.

Becoming Knowledgeable about Stroke

Finally, educate yourself about the symptoms and risks of stroke. However, before you decide to act on any of the information you acquire, keep two precautions in mind. First, *do not self-diagnose*; consult a professional if you are unsure about your symptoms, and before beginning any program or taking any medication. Secondly, *make sure your information comes from a reliable source*. Media documentaries vary in reliability. If their purpose is "investigative reporting" they may be biased toward finding a culprit; if their theme is "progress in science" they may tend to proclaim a breakthrough where none exists. Remember that, for the media, no news is never good news. Even memoirs of stroke victims should be kept in perspective. They often give good insight into what the disease is like from the patient's viewpoint, but remember that all cases are different. The American Heart Association, the Heart and Stroke Foundation of Canada and the National Stroke Association of the United States are the most reliable sources of information.

What about the Internet?
Also be wary of websites containing medical information. The most reliable websites are those of government health agencies, national associations such as the American Heart Association and the Heart and Stroke Foundation of Canada, and top medical centers; they have knowledgeable people who vet the information, and their reports are reliable, updated and helpful. Sites that are supported or produced by advertisers may be more biased, because their primary interest is selling a product or service. Less dependable sites may be misleading and exploitative. Some offer false hopes, and some are real rip-offs, offering "cures" in exchange for cash.

Each person's case is different; that's why it's not a good idea to rely on other people's experiences or testimonials. The best way to gather information about a particular drug or procedure is to look at studies that have scientifically examined its effectiveness. It should be easy to find supportive information for any declarations or facts. Materials from major institutions, or leading publications, especially specialty medical journals, are good sources. On each website you should be able to find the mailing address, contact numbers and credentials of the supporting organization.

Any material claiming a miraculous cure or treatment should be regarded with caution.

Most important, discuss the information you have found with your doctor. Check the reliability of your sources, voice any concerns and discuss any plans for lifestyle change *before* you act on information you have found on the Internet.

TWELVE

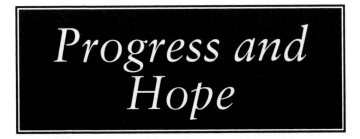

Progress and Hope

In the past quarter of a century the field of stroke, once so full of pessimism and despair, has been lit by new hope, not only for the prevention of stroke but also for successful treatment. Yet, though we have witnessed many advances, breakthroughs take a long time. What may appear to be a stunning advance is in reality the sum of many, many small incremental efforts. It may be hard to believe that anything good can come from a stroke, but it sometimes takes devastation like this to make people focus on what is really important in their lives. The current outlook for stroke patients is better than ever before. Education, research and information are developing rapidly, and creating a future that looks even brighter than the present.

Technical Advances

Imaging
Magnetic resonance techniques (MRI—see Chapter 6) are being refined continuously, and are providing ever more detailed images, not only of the normal and injured brain tissue, but of the blood vessels of the brain.

A number of now experimental MRI techniques may well become routine in the near future. *Magnetic resonance spectroscopy* gives doctors a profile of several important chemicals of

---

Stroke and musical creativity

The Russian composer Shebalin was 57 years of age when he suffered a major stroke affecting his speech areas. He had trouble expressing himself and difficulty understanding what was said to him. Despite this, he continued to compose works that were up to his usual high standard. Dimitri Shostakovitch considered Shebalin's Fifth Symphony, composed after the brain attack, to be "a brilliant creative work." Did the damage to one part of the brain, affecting speech, enhance his musical creativity? We can only guess.

---

the brain, and information about how they change during a stroke.

When part of the brain is used, blood to that area increases slightly. *Functional magnetic resonance imaging* allows us to observe how the brain functions naturally, how it is changed by stroke and how it recovers.

Special techniques using magnetic resonance imaging may show what parts of the brain are injured but still alive; this information can then guide treatment. The imaging revolution will enable doctors to see inside the brain more and more, yet less and less invasively.

The Information Revolution

Doctors continue to make advances in their ability to diagnose stroke, partly because of a growing knowledge base, and partly because of better training and increased access to information. Information can be linked, shared, transferred, transformed and interpreted electronically. For example, in a communication taking mere seconds, information from an MRI scanner can now be sent to a stroke center to be visualized and interpreted. Linkages between university and community hospitals are constantly being increased and extended. This will be extremely beneficial to people who live far from a hospital that has a brain attack unit. With the world connected through the Internet, it's now possible for experts to give a medical consultation almost anywhere.

This is not all good news. It is so easy to set up a website that almost anybody can post almost anything. With growing information, as with anything in bulk, quality suffers. Facts, pseudofacts and outright falsehoods pile up. As noted in Chapter 11, it is important to get information from a reliable source.

The information revolution has made patients better informed. Better-informed patients are more able to help themselves and to be helped. At its best, the Internet offers the inveterate healthcare shopper the opportunity to expand worldwide.

Globalization

Globalization will have an important impact on how stroke is approached. New medications cannot simply be tested in a few developed countries on the assumption that the studies' conclusions will apply everywhere. For example, people from East Asia (such as Chinese, Japanese and Thai) seem more sensitive to drugs that change coagulation, and doses recommended in the West may not be appropriate for them. Involving more countries may speed up research, and may also be more economical. Certainly the conclusions will apply more widely.

New Treatments

Clot-Busting Drugs

After it was demonstrated that the clot-busting drug t-PA could improve a stroke survivor's chance of recovery if given within three hours, researchers began developing other, potentially better types of clot-busting drugs (thrombolytics) that are being tested in clinical trials and have fewer side effects.

Brain-Protective Drugs

When the brain is injured, many things go wrong. A number of drugs that block the steps leading to brain damage are currently being tested on people. For example, glutamate is an important chemical messenger in the brain. When a stroke happens, glutamate spills and damages brain tissue. Several drugs can block this harmful action in animals, but not yet in people.

Combination Treatment

It is likely that in the future a safe brain-protector drug will be given as soon as stroke occurs, in the ambulance or even at home. As soon as bleeding into the head is ruled out by a CT or MRI scan—t-PA could make such bleeding worse—a clot-busting drug will be given, followed by a combination of different brain-protector drugs. Later, drugs that enhance brain recovery will be given, along with a rehabilitation program tailored to the patient.

Treatment Costs

Progress comes at a cost. The more sophisticated the technology or the treatments, the greater the expense. How quickly can the new treatment be applied? Who will pay for it? How cost-effective is it? These questions will be increasingly asked, as both public and private healthcare funding systems come under scrutiny in the United States and Canada.

Scientific and Social Issues

Genetics

If all the risk factors we have discussed were banished from the earth, we would still prevent only half of all strokes. What causes the other half and what we can do about them remains unknown. It is likely that a big part of the answer is genetics—

i.e., what we inherit—and the interaction of genetics with the environment. For example, some people are born prone to obesity, but if they control their diet they may not develop the condition. Genetics sets the limits, but how far you go within those limits depends on your environment, and on you. Genetics already has much to offer, and we are learning more every day about identifying people at risk for brain attack, and about how they will respond to treatment.

Life, Death and the Quality of Life

The older people get, the more healthcare they need. An aging population will inevitably strain the healthcare system, requiring more acute and chronic hospital beds, retirement facilities and nursing homes. Baby boomers are already being caught between helping their not-yet-independent children and helping their dependent parents.

In addition, this aging population is more prone to stroke, thus requiring additional care and services. We can prevent and delay some strokes, but ultimately, until the key to our longevity is found, the best we can hope for is to push disease and death to the outer biological limit, which seems to be about 120 years. We need to take action to prepare for these healthcare demands of the future. Stroke care should be provided in units that cover the spectrum of prevention, treatment, rehabilitation and reintegration into the community. This effective form of organization needs to be implemented more widely.

Looking Forward

The last quarter-century has witnessed tremendous progress in the diagnosis, treatment and prevention of stroke. But although much has been achieved, much more remains to be done. Education about the risk factors and protective factors for stroke, early testing of people who are at risk, and organized and

> ## Did you ever think you would love a snake?
>
> A lot of progress is being made because of innovative research. Recently, doctors in North America showed that an extract of venom from the Malayan pit viper, which can make its victims bleed to death by not allowing their blood to clot, can be used to dissolve blood clots in the brain, if the extract is administered within three hours of the onset of the stroke. These findings await confirmation. The drug has not been approved for general use.

integrated medical care will all help us cope with stroke. So will realism, when someone reaches the point where medical science can do no more.

The next big question that doctors are exploring is "How can we help the brain recover?" Research into how recovery can be enhanced is going forward at an increasing pace—never before have so many advances been made so quickly in understanding how the human body works.

We are also gaining new understanding of how social conditions and the environment relate to human health. Laboratories are yielding answers about basic biological functions at an increasing rate. Doctors are constantly re-evaluating what they do to meet a new high standard: *evidence-based medicine*, which demands proof that what is being advocated or done is effective. You too can play an important part in research—by participating in clinical trials, and by supporting research. Research is our best guarantee of further progress.

Table of Drug Names

Generic Name	Some Brand Names	Action
Stroke Prevention		
Acetylsalicylic acid (ASA)	Bayer Aspirin	prevents blood clots
Clopidogrel	Plavix	prevents blood clots
Dipyridamole	Persantine	prevents blood clots
Dipyridamole plus ASA	Aggrenox	prevents blood clots
Heparin	Heparin	blood thinner
Ticlopidine	Ticlid	prevents blood clots
Warfarin	Coumadin	blood thinner
Stroke Treatment		
Tissue plasminogen activator (t-PA)	Alteplase	re-opens blood vessels

Glossary

Aneurysm: a little blister that bulges from the weakened wall of an artery. If a brain aneurysm ruptures, it causes a subarachnoid hemorrhage.

Antiplatelet drugs: medications that keep small blood cells (platelets) from sticking together, causing clots. Common antiplatelet drugs are acetylsalicylic acid (ASA), ticlopidine, clopidogrel and dipyridamole.

Aphasia: speech disability that may result from stroke. Someone with expressive (Broca's) aphasia cannot express thoughts verbally; someone with receptive (Wernicke's) aphasia cannot understand spoken or written language.

Arterial dissection: tearing apart of the layers of an artery.

Arteriogram: injection of a dye to make pictures of the arteries; *see* **Cerebral angiogram.**

Arteriolosclerosis: disease of the small arteries, usually due to high blood pressure and/or diabetes; *see* **Arteriosclerosis.**

Arteriosclerosis: thickening and loss of elasticity of the walls of arteries, large (atherosclerosis) and small (arteriolosclerosis).

Atherosclerosis: disease of large arteries narrowed by fatty, inflamed, clot-breeding deposits. *See* **Arteriosclerosis.**

Atrial fibrillation: a type of irregular heartbeat that can cause stroke.

Brain attack: a lay term used for stroke and transient ischemic attack, to stress the urgency of getting medical help.

Carotid arteries: the two largest arteries in the neck, which carry most of the brain's blood supply.

Carotid Doppler: measurement of the speed and pattern of blood flow to detect narrowing of the artery; *see* **Ultrasonography.**

Carotid endarterectomy: surgical opening of a narrowing in the main neck artery.

Carotid stenosis: narrowing of a carotid artery.

Cerebral angiogram: injection of dye to make pictures of the neck and brain arteries.

Cerebral infarct: death of a part of the brain due to loss of its blood supply.

Cerebrovascular accident (CVA): stroke.

Cognitive: relating to the ability to think, remember and problem-solve.

Computerized tomography (CT) scan: a special X-ray to show detailed images of the body, e.g. the brain.

CT scan: *see* **Computerized tomography scan.**

CVA: *see* **Cerebrovascular accident.**

Dysarthria: trouble pronouncing words.

Hemiplegia: paralysis of one side of the body.

Hemorrhagic stroke: a stroke due to a burst brain blood vessel. About 20 percent of strokes are hemorrhagic.

High blood pressure: see **Hypertension.**

Hyperhomocysteinemia: abnormal levels of the natural chemical homocysteine in the blood, associated with atherosclerosis.

Hypertension: high blood pressure.

Intracerebral hemorrhage: bleeding into the brain.

Ischemic stroke: a stroke in which the blood supply to part of the brain is blocked, leading to death of brain tissue. About 80 percent of strokes are ischemic.

Magnetic resonance imaging (MRI): noninvasive imaging of the brain using magnetic changes. Functional magnetic resonance imaging shows how well the brain is functioning— after a stroke and during recovery, for example.

Magnetic resonance spectroscopy: a research technique to look at the chemistry of the brain.

MRI: *see* **Magnetic resonance imaging.**

Neurologist: a medical doctor specializing in diseases of the nervous system.

Neurosurgeon: a medical doctor specializing in surgery on the nervous system.

Spasticity: stiffness of a limb resulting from brain or spinal cord damage.

Spatial neglect: lack of awareness on one side, including awareness of the person's own body.

Stroke: loss of function of a part of the brain due to a blocked or burst blood vessel.

Subarachnoid hemorrhage: bleeding around the brain, usually due to a ruptured aneurysm.

Subdural hematoma: a blood clot found between the brain and the skull, usually resulting from trauma to the head.

Thrombolytic drugs: drugs that dissolve blood clots. *See* **Tissue plasminogen activator.**

TIA: *see* **Transient ischemic attack.**

Tissue plasminogen activator (t-PA): a type of clot-busting drug used to treat heart attack and ischemic strokes.

T-PA: *see* **Tissue plasminogen activator.**

Transient ischemic attack: sudden weakness or numbness of the face, arm or leg, loss or slurring of speech, loss or blurring of vision, a sensation of motion, difficulty with balance or a sudden, unusual or severe headache; these symptoms are the same as for a stroke except that they usually go away within minutes. It is still important to get a medical opinion. TIAs are brief brain attacks.

Ultrasonography: the use of sound waves to measure the speed of blood and to create pictures of the blood vessels.

Venous thrombosis: a condition
in which blood clots form in
the veins, usually of the legs
and pelvis; they may travel to
the brain through a hole in the
heart, causing stroke.

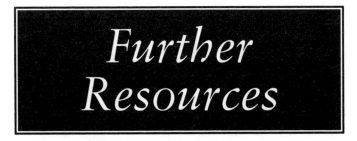

Further Resources

The inclusion of resources is not an endorsement of all their recommendations and is not a substitute for medical advice.

Institutions

U.S.

American Heart Association
7272 Greenville Avenue
Dallas, TX 75231-4596
Toll-free: 1-800-242-8721
www.americanheart.org

American Stroke Association
7272 Greenville Avenue
Dallas TX 75231-4596
Toll-free: 1-888-478-7653
  (U.S. only)
www.strokeassociation.org

Centerwatch
(clinical trials listing service)
22 Thomson Place, 36T1
Boston, MA 02210-1212
(617) 856-5900
www.centerwatch.com

Disability Resource Centre
*(directory of products and
  services)*
jj Marketing
1205 Savoy Street, Suite 101
San Diego, CA 92107
Toll-free: 1-800-787-8444
  (U.S. only)
(619) 222-8735
www.blvd.com

National Family Caregivers
  Association
10400 Connecticut Avenue
Suite 500
Kensington, MD 20895-3944
Toll-free: 1-800-896-3650
(301) 942-6430
www.nfcacares.org

National Institute of
  Neurological Disorders
  and Stroke
Office Building 31, Room 8A16
31 Center Drive
MSC2540
Bethesda, MD 20892
Toll-free: 1-800-352-9424
  (U.S. only)
www.ninds.nih.gov

National Rehabilitation
  Information Center
4200 Forbes Boulevard
Suite 202
Lanham, MD 20706
Toll-free: 1-800-227-0216
  (U.S. only)
(301) 346-2742
www.naric.com

National Stroke Association
9707 E. Easter Lane
Englewood, CO 80112
Toll-free: 1-800-STROKES
(303) 649-9299
www.stroke.org

Society for Accessible Travel
  and Hospitality
347 Fifth Avenue, Suite 610
New York, NY 10016
(212) 447-7284
Fax: (212) 725-8253
www.sath.org

Travelin' Talk Network
P.O. Box 1796
Wheat Ridge, CO 80034
(303) 232-2979
www.travelintalk.net

U.S. Living Will Registry
523 Westfield Avenue
P.O. Box 2789
Westfield, NJ 07091-2789
www.uslivingwillregistry.com

Canada

Accessible Transportation
  Directorate
15 Eddy Street
Hull, PQ K1A 0N9
Toll-free: 1-800-883-1813
www.cta-otc.gc.ca

Association for the
  Neurologically Disabled
  of Canada
59 Clement Road
Toronto, ON M9R 1Y5
Toll-free: 1-800-561-1497
  (outside Toronto)
416-244-1992
www.and.ca

Canadian Association of
  Independent Living Centres
1104–170 Laurier Avenue W.
Ottawa, ON K1P 5V5
(613) 563-2581
Fax: (613) 563-3861
www.cailc.ca

Heart and Stroke Foundation
  of Canada
222 Queen Street, Suite 1402
Ottawa, ON K1P 5V9
(613) 569-4361
Fax: (613) 569-3278
www.heartandstroke.ca

Other Websites

Canadian Health Network
www.canadian-health-network.ca

Healthfinder
www.healthfinder.gov

Mayo Clinic
www.mayohealth.org

National Women's Health Information Center
www.4woman.gov

Stroke Center
www.strokecenter.org

Books

Gordon, Neil F., MD. *Stroke: Your Complete Exercise Guide.* Champaign, IL: Human Kinetics, 1993.

Hayle, Sheila. *The Man Who Lost His Language.* London: Penguin, 2002.

Klein, Bonnie S. *Slow Dance: A Story of Stroke, Love and Disability.* Toronto, ON: Knopf, 1997.

McCrum, Robert. *My Year Off.* Toronto, ON: Knopf, 1998.

Molloy, D.W., MD. *What Are We Going to Do Now?* Toronto, ON: Key Porter, 1996. Published in the United States as *Helping Your Parents in Their Senior Years.* Buffalo, NY: Firefly, 1997.

Senelick, Richard C., MD, Peter W. Rossi, MD, and Karla Dougherty. *Living with Stroke: A Guide for Families.* Chicago, IL: Contemporary, 1999.

Index

Page numbers in italic indicate a figure, table or boxed text. For brand names of medications, please see table p. 125.